Lose Weight with
Dr. Art Ulene

Lose Weight with
Dr. Art Ulene

Art Ulene, M.D.

Ulysses Press
1995

Secrets of Fat-Free Baking, written by Sandra Woodruff, RD, © 1994, 1995. Published by Avery Publishing Group, Inc., Garden City Park, New York. Reprinted by Permission.

Published by: Ulysses Press
P.O. Box 3440
Berkeley, CA 94703-3440

Library of Congress Catalog Card Number: 95-61971

ISBN: 1-56975-048-3

Printed in the USA by the George Banta Company

10 9 8 7 6 5 4 3 2 1

Editor: Laura Golden Bellotti
Cover Design: DesignWorks
Editorial and production staff: Claire Chun, Jennifer Wilkoff, Mark Rosen, Ellen Nidy, Lee Micheaux
Illustrator: Jeannie Brunnick
Indexer: Sayre Van Young
Cover photograph: Michael Helms
Color separation: ProScan, San Carlos, CA

Distributed in the United States by Publishers Group West, in Canada by Raincoast Books, and in Great Britain and Europe by World Leisure Marketing.

Dedication

This book is gratefully dedicated to the TODAY volunteers, from Washington, D.C., who tested this program and shared their triumphs and tribulations with television viewers across the country. They gave up their privacy so that others might be inspired to make healthy lifestyle changes.

CONTENTS

Introduction   1

PART I: OBESITY AS A DISEASE, NOT A HUMAN FAILING   7

   1—A New Theory, A New Experience   9

   2—Understanding Your Weight Regulator   15

   3—Overriding Your Malfunctioning Weight Regulator   25

PART II: TAKING IT OFF, KEEPING IT OFF: THE SCIENCE   33

   4—Lose the Fat, Keep the Muscle   35

   5—Cutting the Fat in Your Diet   39

   6—Increasing Your Physical Activity   45

   7—Modifying Your Eating Behavior   52

   8—Self-Monitoring and Recording Your Progress   57

PART III: TAKING IT OFF, KEEPING IT OFF: THE PROGRAM   75

   9—The Ultimate Goal: Fitness   77

   10—Taking It Off: The Conditioning Phase   83

   11—Taking It Off: The Continuity Phase   241

   12—The Maintenance Phase   310

   Resources   317

   Index   318

ASSIGNMENTS

THE CONDITIONING PHASE

Day 1 90
Day 2 106
Day 3 124
Day 4 139
Day 5 146
Day 6 149
Day 7 157
Day 8 160
Day 9 164
Day 10 168
Day 11 174
Day 12 177
Day 13 181
Day 14 184

Day 15 189
Day 16 195
Day 17 198
Day 18 201
Day 19 204
Day 20 207
Day 21 209
Day 22 213
Day 23 218
Day 24 221
Day 25 224
Day 26 227
Day 27 233
Day 28 240

THE CONTINUITY PHASE

Week 1 271
Week 2 275
Week 3 279
Week 4 283
Week 5 288

Week 6 292
Week 7 298
Week 8 302
Week 9 305
Week 10 308

The author welcomes your comments and questions. He would also appreciate hearing how this book has helped you. Please write to Dr. Art Ulene at P.O. Box 7775, Burbank , CA 91510-7775.

ACKNOWLEDGEMENTS

The author gratefully acknowledges:

- The expertise and inspiration of Arthur Frank, M.D., Medical Director of the George Washington University Obesity Management Program.

- The skillful writing and tireless effort of Richard Trubo.

- The professional contributions and comradeship of Valerie Ulene, M.D.

- The talent, guidance, and endless work of Kukla Vera.

- The valuable contributions of Dana Huebler and Laura Golden Bellotti.

- The administrative efficiency and skill of Jamie McDowell.

- The support of Susan Dutcher and Jeff Zucker, NBC TODAY, who made it possible for us to share this program with millions of viewers.

INTRODUCTION

For 20 years, I've been trying to help overweight people lose their excess pounds. I had a personal interest in the subject because I was always a little overweight myself. But it was my experience as a practicing physician that really made me start to take this issue seriously.

I was a highly trained specialist and saw primarily patients who were referred because of serious medical problems. To my surprise, many of them seemed more troubled about being overweight than about the disorder I was treating them for. Those extra pounds damaged their self-esteem and prompted them to try bizarre and dangerous crash diets. They fasted. They starved. They tried pineapple diets and rice diets. They went to "fat farms." They spent fortunes at commercial weight-loss clinics. Often, these patients did lose weight—in some cases, large amounts. But all too frequently, as soon as they stopped the diets, supplements or drugs they were using, they gained back all of the weight—and then some.

Over the years I developed a healthy respect for the struggles of these people. So when a television producer asked me in 1975 to name two important medical subjects for future programming, I picked weight loss as one of them (breast cancer was the other).

Shortly thereafter, I helped present a series of television reports about weight control on the NBC affiliate in Los Angeles. More than 125,000 viewers "signed up" for our month-long weight-loss program—a simple and safe plan that involved good nutrition and exercise. Station executives estimated that our Los Angeles viewers lost over a million pounds during the series. The program was eventually aired in 50 cities, with the same kind of response and success. I was proud that I could involve so many people in a weight-loss plan that was safe, nutritionally sound, and successful—particularly in view of the frustrations my patients had experienced in past years.

Since then, I have used every available opportunity to educate the public (and myself) about obesity and weight loss. My commitment became even stronger in 1993 when I was exposed to a new and different scientific theory about obesity—one that offered hope of a long-term solution to this problem. You'll learn all about this theory as you read further.

My enthusiasm for the new theory led me to write the book, *TAKE IT OFF! KEEP IT OFF!*, and to air a nationwide, month-long weightloss series on NBC's TODAY show in January of 1995. The response to the book and television reports far exceeded even my most optimistic expectations. More than 12,000 viewers actually sent me their "before" photos when the program started. Millions of viewers followed the series on the air; as best we can determine, literally hundreds of thousands used our program and completed the daily assignments we gave them.

Those daily TV reports on TODAY featured a group of 20 volunteers from the Washington, D.C. area whom we had recruited through newspaper ads in the fall of 1994. They ranged in age from 12 to 70, and their starting weights ranged from 137 to 300 pounds. When they began the program in October, we started videotaping their progress. At that time I nervously joked that if all the volunteers gained weight, my career as a "TV doctor" would be over. We were committed to show their results when the series aired, because NBC News' policy required us to report whatever actually happened, even if all of the volunteers gained weight.

But they didn't gain weight. In fact, they lost a tremendous amount, and as of the time of this writing, most of them are keeping it off! Here's a quick overview of the average weight losses our volunteers experienced:

After 1 month   = 8.5 pounds

After 2 months   = 14.0 pounds

After 3 months   = 19.2 pounds

After 6 months   = 18.5 pounds

When we held a six-month reunion, our volunteers were just as excited about the program as they had been when we began. Suzanne Kraft, a grandmother who had lost 37 pounds, proudly announced that in addition to walking regularly, she had become an occasional jogger, running a mile at a time, and she was still losing weight. Ed Caffery had shed 50 pounds; his general health and energy level had improved so much that his doctor was able to reduce the medications he was taking for asthma and other health problems. Helen Robinson lost 26 pounds, and although she had not been physically active before she joined us, she became an avid walker. You'll meet these and other participants later in this book.

The glowing reports were not limited to our Washington volunteers. Every day, letters and calls poured in from viewers who were using the series to take off weight. A business executive from Louisiana lost 18 pounds in the first 28 days (each morning, he walked up five flights of stairs to his office, and when he traveled on business, he requested hotel rooms on the fifth floor and always used the stairs). A couple from California reported a combined weight loss of 28 pounds in the first few weeks (she lost 21, he lost 7); as a result, her high blood pressure readings came down to normal levels.

A woman from Wisconsin, who dropped her weight from 287 to 266 wrote us, "I can learn to love myself again. It's not too late for me. You have given me hope and a joy for life." Nearly six months after beginning the program, she had lost even more, weighing in at 245 pounds.

A viewer from Delaware, who started our program weighing 208 pounds, described her struggles with high blood pressure and dizzy spells in her initial letter to us. When the TODAY show series began, she threw out the beef, butter, margarine and mayonnaise in her refrigerator. After four months, her blood pressure was down, she had lost 35 pounds, and her husband had lost 40. "We can continue this because it is a lifestyle," she wrote at that four-month point. "I need to lose 30 pounds more—and I will!" And, in fact, she has continued to lose gradually, weighing in at 168 pounds five months after beginning the program.

After all the glowing comments about our weight-loss plan, we were unprepared for the enormous and loud protest we received when the TODAY show series ended after four weeks. People who had more weight to lose complained that we had stopped too soon—leaving them without the additional guidance and motivational support they wanted and needed. Readers of *TAKE IT OFF! KEEP IT OFF!* wanted more than the 28-day program contained in that book.

In response to their comments and suggestions, I have written *LOSE WEIGHT WITH DR. ART ULENE.* This book contains an expanded and improved weight-loss program that incorporates new ideas we learned while implementing the television version of the plan. There are almost 100 pages of new information and illustrations in this book, including some new assignments suggested by viewers and readers, and a new exercise routine designed to protect your muscles as you lose weight. You'll find a new Continuity Phase created for those who still have more weight to lose after 28 days, and extra charts—enough to support six months of weight-loss efforts. And once you weigh just what you want to, our new Maintenance Phase will help you stay there.

The scientific basis of our program is even stronger now. Several major discoveries about obesity that were announced during 1995 have supported our original premise, and helped us understand even more clearly why this program works. You'll read about those breakthroughs, and you'll find new assignments based on recent research.

I hope *LOSE WEIGHT WITH DR. ART ULENE* helps you achieve your weight-loss and fitness goals. But keep in mind that just reading this (or any other) book will not make you lose weight or improve your fitness level (if that were possible, Americans would be the thinnest and fittest people in the world!). You must live the program to reap the benefits. Give it a try. I believe you'll be so pleased with the results that you'll keep it up for a lifetime.

I also hope you'll let me know how you are doing. Write, send photos, and—most important—let me have your suggestions for improving the program. I'll do my best to share your ideas with others.

I wish you good luck and good health always.

Art Ulene, M.D.

PART I
OBESITY AS A DISEASE,
NOT A HUMAN FAILING

1

A NEW THEORY, A NEW EXPERIENCE

Anyone can lose weight. I've done it many times. The trouble is, I never kept it off. For most of my adult life, weight control has been a major issue for me. As a physician and particularly as someone often in the public eye in front of a television camera, I've had to be conscientious about my appearance. I was expected to be a role model for the health-promoting messages I was delivering on television. Even so, I struggled with a weight problem for many years, usually hovering about 15 pounds above my ideal weight. Now and then, I'd lose that excess weight, but every time I'd gain it right back. Frankly, I felt pretty stupid about regaining those pounds, but I didn't seem to be able to do much about it. It was as if some unseen force kept pushing me toward a higher weight, although—as you can readily imagine—I wasn't about to use that excuse to explain my problem to others.

Ironically, during my 20-year career in television, I've reported on obesity dozens of times, and I've investigated an endless stream of weight-loss programs. Most have promised miracles; virtually all fizzle out in the long term. I've interviewed hundreds of frustrated people who dreamed of becoming skinny, but whose dreams were shattered repeatedly by the discouraging reality that weight lost on diets was always regained. I had felt that same frustration myself many times. Why, I wondered, is it so easy to take the weight off, and so difficult to keep it off? Nothing I learned in medical school or in years of doing research for my television series provided an answer—or even an insight.

That changed dramatically in the spring of 1993. One evening, while reading *JAMA* (the *Journal of the American Medical Association*), I came across a commentary that offered a very different perspective on obesity and weight loss. It was written by Dr. Arthur Frank, Medical Director of the George Washington University Obesity Management Program. Dr. Frank argued that it was time to start treating obesity as a chronic disease, not a human failing. In fact, he called obesity "the most common metabolic disease in the United States."

Dr. Frank's explanation of the problem was certainly novel. People do not become fat because they eat too much, he claimed. "A more reasonable analysis," he wrote, "is that, if they overeat, they do so because they have the disease of obesity." This disease, he theorized, upsets your body's weight-regulating mechanism, causing it to establish a new "set point" or weight level that the body then fights to maintain. According to Dr. Frank's theory, it's as if the thermostat on your home furnace accidentally jammed at 90 degrees. You could open the doors and windows to cool things off a little, but that furnace would just keep running until it got the temperature in the house back up to 90 degrees. For the first time, a scientific theory about obesity made sense to me: obesity as a chronic disease, not a human failing.

Dr. Frank's theory explained many of the things that had puzzled me for so long about obesity. For the first time, I could understand those unseen forces that pressured me to regain the weight I lost— again and again. I must confess: Dr. Frank's theory made me feel a lot better about my previous failures at keeping the pounds off.

But I couldn't help wondering whether the theory wasn't just a grand rationalization. Dr. Frank's other comments resolved that issue for me. He pointed out that physicians (and the general public) don't blame people with high blood pressure or diabetes for their problems; yet those chronic diseases are very similar to obesity. Like obesity, both hypertension and diabetes have many different factors that can cause the normal regulating mechanisms to go awry (heredity, diet, exercise, and psychological and environmental issues all may play a role in both diseases). As in obesity, drugs can be used in hypertension and diabetes to adjust the regulating mechanism and reverse the process. As in obesity, if drugs are the only intervention used to treat high blood pressure or high blood sugar, the problem will return as soon as the drug therapy is stopped. As with obesity, a person with hypertension or diabetes can make relatively straightforward lifestyle changes to override the abnormal regulating system and reverse the disease process. And finally, like obesity, both hypertension and diabetes are chronic, lifelong conditions—and they must be treated as such.

Although Dr. Frank's ideas about a weight regulator that had gone awry appealed to me, the concept was still difficult to accept. After all, no one, including Dr. Frank, could show me where the regulator was actually located (it's really hard to shake off the constraints that the anatomy lab puts on your thinking). And even Dr. Frank couldn't explain in his commentary precisely how the regulator worked. He described the weight regulator as a complex mechanism that somehow took into account all of the forces that influence our weight, including heredity, diet, eating behaviors, hormones, enzymes, and exercise. "Somehow," he observed, "the forces are orchestrated to sustain a beautiful symphony in normal-weight people and chaotic dissonance in people with the disease of obesity." That description was more poetic than scientific, but it was consistent with many other observations about how the human body works (or breaks down), and it seemed logical to me.

I was so intrigued and excited by Dr. Frank's commentary in *JAMA* that I wrote to him, and that letter led to a series of phone conversations between us. Before long, I began to test some of his ideas on myself. This time my experience with weight loss was different.

Not only did the weight come off—it stayed off. Better yet, this time there was no struggle, no sense of deprivation, and within a few weeks, almost no effort. This time, when I felt those overpowering and self-defeating urges to eat poorly or skip my regular exercise routine, I recognized them as my weight regulator's attempt to return to the weight that it was programmed to maintain.

I must confess, my weight-loss routine was very different from the routines I had tried before. I ate more and enjoyed the food more. In the past I had skipped meals. This time I ate three meals plus two snacks a day. Previously I had exercised at very high intensity once or twice a week. This time I slowed to a walk, but did it every day. For the first time in my life, I actually enjoyed exercise. In the past, I weighed myself three or four times a day. This time, I used the scale three or four times a week and stopped worrying about the result.

As I write this book, the 15 extra pounds are gone, and I have no worry about their returning. My fitness level has improved so dramatically that, for the first time, I look forward to running in the morning, I lead the pack in weekend bike rides, and my resting heart rate has dipped to an extremely healthy 52 beats a minute. I've never felt better!

A Program for Lasting Weight Loss

This book has grown out of my need to share these ideas with you. In the pages that follow, I will introduce you to what I have learned, and explain how you can use this information to have lasting success, too. You'll read about the causes of obesity and the factors that influence the activity of your internal weight regulator. Then we'll give you a program to help you take control of your weight regulator—not just to lose weight, but to keep it off, comfortably, for the rest of your life.

Our program is not a diet, because diets don't work. Although diets can produce weight loss, they also create feelings of deprivation that lead to rebound eating and weight gain. Diets are too rigid for today's busy schedules and lifestyles. And, by definition, anyone who goes on a diet must ultimately go off it. You know what happens then.

So you will find no rigid menus or meal plans, no forbidden foods, no calorie counting, and no meal substitutes (liquid lunch in a can is not acceptable to me, so I could not recommend it to you). Instead, we'll show you how several small changes in food selection and eating behavior, combined with small (but significant) incremental increases in your activity level, can help you override a weight regulator that is frustrating your attempts to keep the lost pounds off. You'll learn how to recognize and neutralize those unseen forces that have been controlling your behavior in the past. Slowly but surely, you'll gain control over your weight regulator, instead of letting it control you.

Believe it or not, if you follow our program faithfully, you'll not only lose weight, you'll learn to enjoy the process. Sound far-fetched? I used to love the feel and flavor of fat in everything I ate. Now I can't even drink whole milk or eat regular yogurt—they taste too rich. I used to routinely skip meals and race through the ones I ate. But I've adjusted my priorities. Now, I eat three meals a day, and I take time to enjoy them. I used to hate exercise. I rarely miss a day now because I don't feel right anymore if I don't get some physical activity. (To be perfectly honest, I still hate getting out of bed to begin exercising, but I now know that this is my weight regulator's way of trying to reverse my success and get my weight back up where it was.) I used to feel controlled by my scale, and spent too much time criticizing myself when I gained a pound or two. Now the scale is my friend. It helped me measure my progress while I was losing weight, and it reminds me now how easy it is to gain back those pounds if I let my weight regulator take control of my behavior again.

You can learn how to make these kinds of changes, too. By adopting the highly effective techniques I will show you, you can learn how to enjoy the process of weight loss, and you can condition your mind and body to do it effortlessly. That's a promise—if you follow the program precisely as it is described in this book.

A Program for Life, Not a Diet

If you are like most people reading this book, chances are you're an expert on weight cycling and diets. You've lost weight several times and gained it all back—and then some. The chances are even greater that you're skeptical about finding a program that will work for you in the long term.

But in the pages that follow, we'll show you a program that's different from any diet you've ever tried. This program combines the unique and effective techniques that Dr. Frank has developed for his obesity clinic at George Washington University Medical School, with the information I have gained from my television viewers and readers over the years. This program will teach you how to override your weight regulator's attempts to drive your weight to the higher set point it has chosen for you. It will deal in a systematic and synergistic manner with the major weight-promoting factors that are susceptible to change (we can't do anything about the genetic tendencies you've inherited).

The program will also help you make several changes in the way you think and act. Although we'll introduce these changes gradually, you may find that the first few days of the program require a bit of concentration and effort. That's normal, because any kind of change is difficult for most of us. But I can promise you this: If you follow our 28-day Conditioning Phase program to the letter, you will literally recondition your weight-regulating process so you can begin to take pounds off automatically and almost effortlessly. As a result of this reconditioning process, rather than relying on conscious deprivation and willpower, as most weight-loss diets require you to do, you will develop a subconscious mind-set that supports your goals and makes every weight-loss action easier.

2

UNDERSTANDING YOUR
WEIGHT REGULATOR

Throughout the day, finely tuned regulating systems are hard at work within your body. They govern everything from the regular beating of your heart to the complex workings of your digestive system. When they function well, these regulators keep you healthy, without your even being aware of their existence or how crucial they are to your well-being.

Thanks to modern science, we have a clear understanding of the way most of these regulating systems operate—and what happens when they go awry. Consider, for instance, the physiological system for regulating the hormone insulin, which is produced by the pancreas. Insulin is essential for managing your body's use of glucose, the simple sugar that the body's cells require to carry out many of their activities. But some people do not produce enough insulin, or their bodies do not use it efficiently. As a result, their system for regulating sugar is defective, and dangerous levels of sugar build up in the blood, producing the disease we know as diabetes. Some diabetics may require insulin to restore the system to working order, but others can override the defective regulator and manage their disease process by eating better, becoming more physically active, and maintaining normal body weight.

The same is true with hypertension, or high blood pressure, which requires the heart to work harder than normal to pump blood and oxygen throughout the body. In most cases of hypertension, doctors do not understand why the blood pressure regulatory system goes so far out of kilter. Nevertheless, 50 to 75 percent of people with high blood pressure are able to override the malfunctioning regulator and regain control of their blood pressure without medication, by changing their diets (particularly cutting back on salt intake), increasing their physical activity, losing excess weight, and managing stress more effectively.

Obesity As a Disease

We now believe that, in many ways, obesity is a similar type of chronic disorder, caused by a malfunctioning of the regulatory system that determines your weight. For decades, we've presumed that overweight people just eat too much. Now, we have reason to think that obesity is a disorder in its own right, propelled by disruptions in a complex regulator that determines the "set point" at which your body will try to keep your weight. Driven by powerful internal forces, this weight regulator keeps you heavier than you would like to be—month after month, year after year. And every time you diet and lose some weight, the regulator pressures you to put it back on until you reach the elevated level at which it is set.

A series of studies at the University of Rochester has demonstrated just how powerful this disease process is. Obese individuals were prescribed weight-loss medications for periods as long as three and a half years. These medications worked in the brain at a biological level, influencing chemicals that control eating behavior. During this lengthy time, the drugs overpowered the weight regulator and helped these people lose substantial amounts of weight. But after the pills were withdrawn, even after years of having maintained normal weight, people in the study regained the lost pounds. When their bodies' regulatory forces were no longer restrained with medication, their weight was propelled right back up to the levels determined by their malfunctioning weight-regulating systems.

What does the weight regulator look like? I'd like to be able to point to a single structure in your brain or a single organ in your body and say, "This is what's pushing your weight to high levels." In fact, though, we have not yet been able to identify a single structure in the body that performs this function. Instead, the weight regulator seems to be a complex network of biological mechanisms, genetic factors, and psychological and environmental forces that interact with one another. When all of these elements are working together properly, the regulator automatically keeps your weight at precisely the right level. But when this system malfunctions, a higher set point is established. From then on, the malfunctioning regulator keeps pressuring your body to maintain your weight at that higher level.

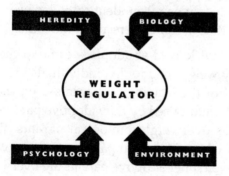

The Factors That Influence Your Weight Regulator

We are just starting to appreciate the complex interactions influencing the set point that the weight regulator selects. In some people, genetics may be the overriding force. In others, biological factors (such as brain chemicals or enzymes) may assume the primary role. In still other individuals, the weight regulator has broken down for reasons that aren't clear. Most often, several of these influences seem to be working together, pushing the regulator toward a high set point, and pressuring you to maintain a higher weight than you desire.

Let's look more closely at the elements that contribute to obesity, and that collectively determine the set point your regulator will choose.

HEREDITY

In a real sense, obesity is a family disease. Studies show that, for 30 to 50 percent of people who are overweight, a significant hereditary component is at work—a genetic destiny that makes them more susceptible to obesity. If a tendency to be overweight runs in your family, you have a greater chance of being overweight.

How powerful are these genetic forces? Studies of twins and adoptees show that when it comes to obesity, heredity is a more important factor than environment. Researchers have found that identical twins—who share common genes—tend to have very similar weight patterns, whether they grow up in the same or different households. Even when identical twins were raised by separate families, their weights were about the same.

Other studies that looked at adoptees came to the same conclusion. The body weight of adopted individuals was closely associated with that of their biological parents—not the parents who raised them. A child raised by thin adoptive parents is likely to be obese if he has overweight biological parents. Conversely, an adopted child whose biological parents are thin will probably be thin himself, even if her adoptive parents are overweight.

Many investigators now believe that although an individual's genes determine whether he or she may tend to become obese, other factors determine whether the individual will in fact become overweight, and just how serious the weight problem will be.

BIOLOGICAL FACTORS

Many biological factors can influence whether or not a person who is susceptible to obesity will actually become obese. These

OBESITY GENES

The genetic influence on obesity is not easy to pin down. While a single gene determines whether you have blue eyes or brown, many genes probably contribute to obesity. In the last year, researchers have made tremendous progress in identifying how some of these genetic influences work.

The most notable achievement was made by a group of investigators at Rockefeller University, who discovered what is probably one of the most important parts of the genetic control of body weight—an "obesity gene" in mice. The gene encodes a protein— called leptin—which researchers believe works by telling the brain how much fat is stored in adipose tissues. When normal and obese mice were compared, the obese mice were found to produce abnormal leptin, or not to produce leptin at all. It is thought that these mice consume excessive amounts of food because their brain never receives a message that they have enough fat stored, which would signal the brain to send messages to "stop eating."

When a group of obese mice (all of whom had an abnormal obesity gene) were treated with daily injections of leptin, they lost an average of 30 percent of their body weight in just two weeks. For comparison, another group of obese mice were offered an identical diet but did not receive leptin; rather than losing weight, they rapidly gained massive amounts of body fat.

Researchers feel that the leptin injections ultimately resulted in satiety signals that had been lacking in the mice, thereby curbing their appetite (the leptin-treated mice ate less). Interestingly, the mice given leptin also became more physically active, suggesting that this protein may help regulate body fat in a number of different ways.

The situation is undoubtedly more complex in humans than in mice. However, a gene similar to the obesity gene in mice has been identified in humans, and studies are currently under way to determine if defects in this gene could be responsible for creating (or at least contributing to) weight-control problems in humans.

include brain chemicals, the quantity of fat cells in the body, the activity level of fat storage enzymes, the person's resting metabolic rate, hormone levels, fidgeting, and thermogenesis. Many of these factors are beyond our control. Others, however, can be influenced by our own actions and behavior.

Brain chemicals. Natural substances called endorphins are foremost among the chemicals that exert strong influences upon your eating behavior. The brain produces hundreds of different endorphins, which are involved in processes ranging from pain perception to blood pressure regulation. Probably several dozen of them play a role in eating behavior. The level and activity of these endorphins are responsive to a number of influences, including when and what you last ate and your activity level. Abnormal levels of these endorphins can signal you to continue eating even after you have had as much food as you need—much to the detriment of your efforts to control your weight. Although the complexity of these endorphins generally leaves them beyond your control, medications prescribed for weight loss may be able to influence them.

Fat cells. The number of fat cells in the body is an important factor in obesity. Whereas a person of normal weight has 25 to 35 billion fat cells, a person who is extremely obese may have 50 to 150 billion, each one capable of storing fat. During periods of weight gain, fat cells can grow dramatically in size, with their diameters multiplying as much as 20 times.

Your number of fat cells is generally beyond your control. When you lose weight, you deplete these fat cells, but you can never get rid of them. Some researchers believe that when you lose weight, shrinking fat cells begin sending out signals to the brain to warn of "starvation"—signals that in turn trigger messages from the brain that create urges to eat.

Fat storage. An enzyme called lipoprotein lipase has a crucial biological influence upon your weight. This enzyme is responsible for moving fat from the bloodstream into storage within the body, essentially playing the role of a gatekeeper. If you are overweight, this enzyme may be functioning too efficiently in encouraging fat storage.

There is some evidence that cigarette smoking may actually suppress lipoprotein lipase. One theory about the role of smoking in keeping weight down is that chemicals in the cigarette smoke destroy lipoprotein lipase and thus interfere with the body's efficient storage of fat. Of course, extraordinary health hazards are also associated with smoking, and it could never be justified as a means of controlling weight.

Resting metabolic rate. No matter how physically inactive you are, your body burns calories just to stay alive. It needs this energy to maintain the function of vital organs such as your brain, heart, liver, lungs, and kidneys. The number of calories an individual burns while at rest is called the resting (or basal) metabolic rate (RMR or BMR). The resting metabolic rate accounts for about 60 to 70 percent of the calories an average person burns each day.

However, the resting metabolic rate can vary considerably from one person to another. In general, large people tend to burn more calories than smaller people. And people with large muscles burn calories faster than people of equal weight, but with a larger proportion of body fat. A 5'10", 170-pound man with a lean and muscular physique will thus use up more calories just by sitting still than will a 5'1" obese woman who weighs 170. That's one reason why the pounds you lose should come from the fat in your body, not the muscle.

The rate at which your body burns calories when it is at rest plays an important part in determining your body weight. The slower your metabolism, the fewer calories you burn, and the more difficulty you'll have controlling your weight. If you burn 2,000 calories a day, you'll have an easier time controlling it than someone who burns 1,500 calories a day. If you're overweight, your resting metabolic rate may be lower than that of normal-weight people.

Thermogenesis. The body uses a biological process called thermogenesis to get rid of excess calories. In this process, some unneeded calories are expended by converting them into heat. Thermogenesis is responsible for about 10 percent of the calories an average person burns each day. Thermogenesis is a factor that affects your weight, but it's an internal process you can't consciously control.

Thus, just as you can't change your resting metabolic rate (except for a short time after exercising, or by building more lean muscle tissue), you can't consciously change your body's rate of thermogenesis. Although thermogenesis probably works quite efficiently in most people of normal weight, the process works less effectively in some overweight individuals. In these people, it may be one of the factors contributing to the breakdown of the weight-regulating system, predisposing them to obesity.

Physical activity. Any muscular activity increases the rate at which you burn calories. The more vigorous the activity, the more calories will be burned. Later in this book, I'll discuss deliberate physical activity such as exercise, and the impact it can have on weight management. But it's important to be aware that some physical activity occurs without conscious thought, and is called fidgeting.

Fidgeting is a random, purposeless activity, and it tends to run in families. Because it's done unconsciously, people who fidget aren't even aware of it. They bounce their leg, tap their fingers, or walk aimlessly around the room. Exasperated by such activity in their children, parents are often heard to exclaim, "Don't fidget!" But calories are burned during fidgeting; so ironically, this often annoying behavior can actually contribute to weight loss.

Through fidgeting, the average person burns about 300 calories a day—about what you'd burn in an hour of brisk walking. But people vary widely in the number of calories they burn through fidgeting. Some people fidget away as few as 100 calories a day; others lose as many as 800 calories a day by fidgeting. But even a 100-calorie loss per day is the equivalent of ten pounds of weight loss per year.

Hormones. Hormones play a role in fat storage. In very complex ways, thyroid hormones, growth hormones, and insulin help regulate storage of fat. In particular, abnormal insulin levels can wreak havoc with your body's metabolism and interfere with the mechanism for keeping your weight normal.

For years, the thyroid shouldered much of the blame for physiological changes that contribute to obesity. Now, however, we know that this small gland, located in the neck, is just one of many elements that can be involved in obesity. The thyroid probably makes a significant contribution in only a small number of cases. In fact, taking thyroid replacement medications is useless except in those cases where significant thyroid underactivity has been documented by laboratory tests.

PSYCHOLOGICAL ISSUES

People eat for lots of reasons that have nothing to do with hunger. In fact, in our culture, where food is plentiful, hunger tends to play only a small role in eating for many individuals. People may turn to food because they're tired, bored, lonely, angry, anxious, stressed, or depressed. Food is also an important part of socializing, entertaining, and celebrating. In some families, food is used to demonstrate love. People who grow up in such families may still reach for food whenever they feel the need for affection. Unfortunately, all they accomplish is to consume calories they don't need, because no amount of food can really satisfy their emotional hunger.

To make matters worse, profound psychological consequences are associated with being overweight. Obese individuals often feel ashamed of their appearance and their supposed lack of willpower. If they try dieting but later regain the lost weight, their morale and sense of hope can be destroyed, further interfering with their ability to gain control of their obesity.

ENVIRONMENTAL ISSUES

Environmental factors can also significantly influence your internal weight regulator. In addition to acquiring a hereditary predisposition to obesity from your parents, you may also have adopted their eating behaviors and their preferences for food. If you were raised in a family of rapid eaters or overeaters, you may eat too much or too rapidly now. If you were raised on high-fat meals and were never exposed to high-fiber, vegetable-rich dining, you are more likely to continue choosing high-fat dishes as an adult. If your family members routinely took second and third helpings, you may have become accustomed to doing so, too. You also may have learned to respond more to the sight and smell of food, rather than to internal sensations of hunger.

Environmental factors like these can be strong influences that sabotage the normal functioning of your weight regulator. People with a healthy weight-regulating system find it relatively easy to close the refrigerator door or walk past the doughnut shop when they are not truly hungry. But under the same circumstances, those with the disease of obesity may feel literally compelled to eat. Usually they have no awareness of the internal forces driving them to eat and, therefore, no understanding of the real reasons they do so.

It's a relief to learn that a weight-regulating system exists in your body—even if it is working against your efforts to control your weight. For one thing, knowing about the weight regulator helps alleviate some of the guilt and shame that overweight people often feel because of the widespread assumption that they are simply paying the price for their own gluttony and laziness. The weight regulator also provides a logical explanation for the mysterious urges, cravings, and behaviors that make it so difficult to keep weight off after it is lost. In the next chapter, I'll show you what you can do to control your weight regulator if it is not functioning properly.

3

OVERRIDING YOUR MALFUNCTIONING WEIGHT REGULATOR

Even though we cannot actually point to a physical structure we can identify as the weight-regulating system, your body operates as though one existed. And when this system malfunctions and moves your "set point" to a higher level, your weight will tend to stay at that level for life. That is why some people stay 20 pounds overweight throughout their life, while others stabilize at weights that are 40 or 60 or 80 pounds above their ideal level. If gaining excess weight were simply a matter of eating too much or being too sedentary, all of these people would be adding pounds continuously throughout their life.

But even if you have a malfunctioning weight regulator, you can still lose weight, because there are many ways to "overpower" the regulator. For example, you can lose weight by starving yourself or by following a diet that severely restricts your caloric and nutritional intake. However, once you start eating normally again, the weight comes back. That is precisely what happens to most people who lose weight this way, because the drastic dietary changes cannot be tolerated for long periods, and the nutritional deficiencies they create are too dangerous.

That's why we have chosen a different approach for overriding your weight regulator, an approach you can use for a lifetime. It combines the ease and effectiveness of small changes and the efficiency of variety with the power of time to create a program you can live with safely and comfortably. This approach will help you lose fat instead of muscle. It will produce not only weight loss, but fitness. It is the right approach to use when you really care about your health.

Making Small Changes Work for You

With most diets and weight-loss plans, large changes are made to produce rapid weight loss. But large changes are difficult to tolerate and sustain, and they produce rapid weight loss at the expense of lean muscle tissues. So our plan relies on small changes that are easy to tolerate. You will soon see what a big difference these small changes can make in your weight when you maintain them over time.

If you have a lot of weight to lose, you may be wondering if small changes are still appropriate in your case. Perhaps these few examples will help convince you how effective this approach can be:

- If you switch from three glasses of whole milk each day to three glasses of skim milk, you will leave 22 pounds of fat behind every year.

- By putting a tablespoon of mustard on your sandwich each day in place of a tablespoon of mayonnaise, you could lose about nine pounds a year.

- Switch from 2 percent fat cottage cheese to dry curd cottage cheese—1 cup a day, four times a week—and you could lose four and a half pounds a year.

- Just one peanut a day adds up to a quarter-pound in three months.

Putting Time on Your Side

With most diets and weight-loss plans, time is your enemy. The longer you follow these plans, the more deprived you feel. The program you are starting now will turn time into an ally. As you slow your eating pace, you'll gain new control over food. Time will help you with exercise, too, as the conditioning effect takes hold and your fitness level begins to increase. And the longer you use our program, the more natural and comfortable your new behaviors will feel to you. Here are some examples that demonstrate the power of time:

- Walk one mile a day and you will lose about ten pounds in a year.

- Eat 1 cup of corn flakes, instead of 1 cup of plain natural granola, three mornings a week, and you could lose 19 pounds in a year.

- Substitute 1 cup of orange sherbet for 1 cup of premium ice cream twice a week, and you could lose almost four pounds in a year.

- Skip just one peanut a day for ten years and you will save ten pounds.

Using Variety to Increase Your Efficiency

Many diets and weight-loss plans focus intensely on a single area of nutrition or activity to produce their results, sometimes taking the process to bizarre and dangerous extremes. This approach has led to such strange things as an ice cream diet, a pineapple diet, a rice diet—even a champagne diet. It's a great way to sell books, but a dangerous way to lose weight.

The program described in this book uses a variety of activities and behaviors to attack your weight-regulating problem from different directions simultaneously. You will cut the amount of fat you eat, increase your physical activity, slow your eating speed, reduce your reactive eating (I'll explain that on page 150), build a support system, and chart your progress. Even if you slip with one of these activities, the others will "cover" you. And if you do all of them every day, you can achieve dramatic results. For example, just cut out one ounce of fat, walk two miles, and leave a few bites of food on your plate every day and you'll lose 66 pounds in a year.

Other Issues That Influence Weight Loss

Several other issues can influence the long-term success of your weight-loss program.

Motivation. Your desire to lose weight is a crucial element in your ultimate success. I've found that most dieters are actually very well motivated, particularly in the early days of their weight-loss efforts. Many are trying to lose weight to improve their appearance. Some believe that weight loss will contribute to their success and acceptance on the job. Others hope it will improve their social and sexual life.

Some people, however, begin their weight-loss program with the wrong motivation for success. They've been pressured by a spouse ("I'm embarrassed to be seen with you"). Or they've been pushed into a program by a doctor who failed to spend enough time discussing the health risks of obesity. These people tend to be poorly motivated, and they generally either fail to lose weight, or lose weight but put it right back on.

Sex and Age. Studies show that men are more successful in their weight-loss efforts than women, for reasons that aren't fully understood. In general, men do lose weight more easily, at least in part because they have more lean tissue, pound for pound, than women. This lean tissue plays an important role in determining a person's metabolic rate and consequently in weight loss. For the same reason, younger people tend to lose weight more easily than older ones. For instance, a 30-year-old woman will probably have less difficulty shedding her excess weight than a 50-year-old woman, if they are of comparable size. Again, that's because usually the younger woman will have more lean tissue, her metabolic rate will be higher, and her fat-burning mechanism will be more efficient.

One other point: Although men are more likely to lose weight than women, and to lose it faster, some research indicates that they are less likely to maintain their losses. The reason may be that men are often less willing to deal with the psychological issues that may contribute to their obesity. As one man once said to me, "Don't bother me with all the psychological stuff; I just want to lose weight."

Medical Issues. On occasion, illness itself can interfere with a weight-loss program—for instance, people with severe arthritis may sometimes find it difficult to increase their level of physical activity. However, that same physical pain can also turn into a strong motivator. When you're hurting, you might become that much more dedicated to ridding yourself of excess weight that is contributing to your discomfort.

Degree and Duration of Obesity. Although you might think that people with lots of weight to lose are more likely to fail on diets, they often turn out to be more desperate, more motivated, and more understanding of their need to make long-term changes. By contrast, even though individuals who are trying to lose only 10 or 15 pounds have much less of a challenge ahead of them, they tend to be less willing to make a commitment to the steps they must take to later maintain that weight loss, so their weight regulator keeps tugging them back up to their starting points.

What about men and women who have been obese for many years or even decades? They clearly have a more serious illness than those who have been overweight for just a year or two, and their obesity has probably had a more severe impact on their lives. These people may have experienced many more adverse health consequences from being overweight. The behaviors that contribute to their excess weight have also become more solidly established. Nevertheless, people who have had lengthy histories of obesity tend to be more sensitive to the impact that obesity has had upon their lives, and they are more realistic about what they need to do to finally get their weight under control. They recognize that they're going to have to make major changes in their lifestyles.

Incidentally, if you've failed on diets many times before, that's generally a bad sign for your chances of future success using ordinary diets. But I know of many exceptions to this rule, and your chances of success with the very different, non-diet approach you are about to try should be just as good as anyone else's. One of our greatest success stories involves a couple who lost a combined total of 167 pounds (she lost 107, he lost 60). This couple had failed again and again over many years with conventional diets and commercial diet programs and products. The message? Even if you've failed ten times in your past efforts to lose weight, you can still succeed on your eleventh try.

Social and Family Support. If your friends or family members are supporting your efforts to lose weight, consider yourself very fortunate. Your chances of success are much higher if you exercise regularly with a friend or family member, or if other members of your household are willing to make changes—for instance, by keeping tempting high-fat foods out of the house. One of the best things you can do if you live with others is to ask for their help as you begin this program.

Too often, however, the people who should be providing support assume the role of saboteur. Family members may be indifferent to your dieting efforts, or—even worse—they'll insist on keeping your trigger foods in the house, and even challenge your resolve ("C'mon, don't make me eat this cake all by myself; how much harm can one slice do?"). They might have an agenda of their own, like the spouse who fears that if his wife loses weight, she will become more attractive to other men and he may lose her. Family members may be quite content with the status quo, even if it means undermining the weight-loss program of the person they claim to love.

Incidentally, as helpful as support groups can be for some people, other dieters fare quite well on their own. In fact, when people responded to our TODAY show weight-loss survey a few years ago, the most successful people had shed their extra weight on their own, concentrating on dietary changes, exercise, and behavior modification techniques, without the help of organized groups or weight-loss products.

Staying Realistic

As you begin this program, keep in mind that your initial weight loss may not be as dramatic with our approach as with other weight-loss plans or diets you've tried or heard advertised. That's because we put your safety and health first—ahead of rapid weight loss. So don't be disappointed if you lose weight more slowly than you've experienced with other diet programs, or more slowly than the wild promises that are being made in newspaper ads and television infomercials. Your weight loss may be gradual, but it will be steady and safe. Stick with this approach and you will not only lose weight, but feel healthier, too.

Now let's get started.

PART II
TAKING IT OFF,
KEEPING IT OFF:
THE SCIENCE

4

LOSE THE FAT,
KEEP THE MUSCLE

Which would you rather lose: fat or muscle? That may sound like a silly question, but research shows that many—if not most—diets cause people to lose weight from their muscles and other lean body tissues at the same time they are losing fat. That's how the body reacts when caloric intake is cut back too drastically.

The more severely you restrict your intake of calories, the more your weight loss will come from muscle instead of fat. During semistarvation, the lean tissue loss can rise to as high as 70 percent of the total weight lost (which means that seven out of every ten pounds you lose are from lean tissue like muscle and only three are from fat!). With moderate caloric restriction, on the other hand, losses of lean body tissue weight can be as little as 15 percent of your total weight loss.

A weight-loss program that causes your muscle tissues to deteriorate will make you lose more than just weight. You'll lose much of your strength, too. Protecting your muscles and confining your

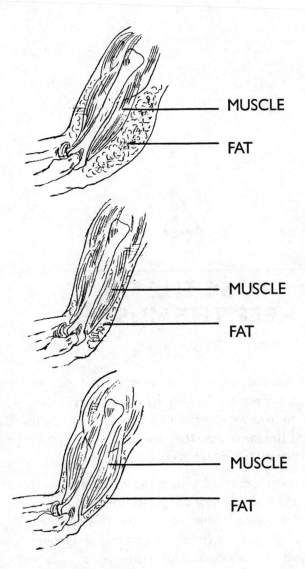

MUSCLE

FAT

MUSCLE

FAT

MUSCLE

FAT

The amount of fat and muscle in your arms (and elsewhere in your body) will vary, depending on the type of weight-loss and exercise strategies you choose. The first diagram depicts the arm of an overweight person prior to beginning a weight-loss program; it has much more fat than muscle. The second drawing shows the arm after the individual has adopted a program of caloric restriction, without exercise; the arm has lost not only fat, but also muscle. The final diagram depicts the same arm, but this time following a program of both caloric reduction and exercise; the arm has lost fat, but it has maintained and even gained a small amount of muscle tissue.

weight loss as much to fat as possible is important for other reasons, too. Losing fat enhances the health benefits of weight loss. It reduces your risk of heart disease and stroke, and decreases your chances of developing hypertension and certain forms of cancer. Losing lean body tissues like muscle, on the other hand, provides none of these benefits.

Protecting your muscle mass will improve your appearance, as well. Building muscles while you lose the surrounding fatty tissue will provide you with good "tone" and "definition," which are responsible for the natural curves and youthful appearance of people who are in good condition.

Losing muscle tissue will not only damage your health—it will hinder your weight-loss efforts. That's because muscle is metabolically active—far more active than other tissues—especially more active than fat. Muscles burn more calories than other tissues when you are resting. When you are active, the difference is even greater, because more energy is required by the muscles when they are working, while fatty tissues have essentially no work to do.

When you lose muscle instead of fat, you decrease the number of calories your body will burn in the future. So, when you are losing weight, it's critical to lose the weight from fat and protect your muscle as much as possible. This may sound obvious, but that is not what happens with most weight-loss diets, which achieve their weight loss solely through caloric restriction. On many of these diets, when you take off five pounds, only two or three of them are from fat—the rest comes from lean tissue. The damage to muscle tissue is even greater on diets that involve fasting or severe restriction of protein or carbohydrates.

How do you increase the proportion of your body that is lean tissue and decrease the proportion that is fat? Very simply—you increase the activity in your daily life at the same time as you decrease the fat in your diet. That is precisely the plan you will follow in our program. It will give you a tremendous advantage over traditional diets that focus only on cutting calories.

One other important point should be made about fat versus lean muscle mass. Muscle tissue is heavier and denser than fat. As you follow this program, you will be losing fat and rebuilding muscle, so don't be surprised if you find yourself losing weight at a slower pace initially than you have experienced on diets that severely restricted caloric intake and caused muscle destruction.

Even though it may not register as clearly on the bathroom scale, your fat loss will be noticeably apparent in a full-length mirror, where you can see the inches you are losing. As you lose excess fat and tone your muscles, you'll notice your body becoming leaner, firmer, and stronger. This visual feedback and the numbers on your tape measurement are better indicators of fat reduction and fitness level than the bathroom scale. Be assured that if you follow our program, you will lose both weight and inches—primarily from fat.

You will also notice a marked improvement in your sense of well-being—your overall attitude and the way you feel about your body. You will feel physically better in a lean, strong, and healthy body, and you will also enjoy the sense of accomplishment and achievement that comes from finally feeling in control of your weight. Feeling physically and psychologically better, and rewarded by positive feedback from your mirror and tape measure (and from family and friends), you will be more motivated to continue your efforts at weight control—making it easier to resist the upward pressure exerted by your weight regulator.

If you are concerned that starting an exercise program will only increase your already active appetite, we have good news for you. In theory, your concern makes sense. The more energy you expend, the more food energy you'll need to replace it. However, studies show that the energy intake of obese people is not significantly increased when they initiate an exercise program. (Normal-weight people, on the other hand, tend to eat more when they increase exercise levels.) In fact, many obese people who exercise say that their appetite actually decreases. After trying our program, we think you'll say the same thing.

5

CUTTING THE FAT
IN YOUR DIET

For decades, the emphasis in weight loss was on cutting calories at any cost. This focus gave rise to a host of eating plans that often were no better than starvation diets. It also produced an array of diet products that were extremely low-calorie substitutes for "real" food. Although these diet programs and products could produce short-term weight loss, they rarely worked over the long term. These very low-calorie plans left people feeling deprived, so as soon as they went off the diet, they quickly resumed their old eating patterns and just as quickly regained their lost weight.

Now it appears that while calories do count, they are not the most important issue for a weight-loss program; dietary fat is. Even though we are bombarded with advertisements proclaiming the array of foods that are "low fat" or "fat free," the American diet is still one of the fattiest in the world. The average adult gets about 37 percent of total calories from fat, nearly double the fat intake we recommend in this program. Cutting back on fat is one of the best mechanisms for overriding your weight regulator. In fact, research shows that cutting your intake of dietary fat is perhaps the easiest and most effective way to lose excess fat on your body, and keep it off over the long term. Let's look at what some recent studies have shown.

In research at Cornell University, 13 women were placed on either a reduced-fat diet (with 20 to 25 percent of their calories coming from fat) or a high-fat diet (with 35 to 40 percent of calories from fat). Neither group of women, however, was asked to limit the number of calories they consumed, and thus they were free to choose the portion sizes they preferred.

After 11 weeks on their assigned diets, each group of women switched to the other diet: Those on the low-fat plan switched to the high-fat one, and vice versa. At the end of the study, the doctors conducting the research found that while on the reduced-fat diet, the women not only ate fewer calories, but lost twice as much weight as they did when eating the high-fat diet. As the investigators observed, "These results demonstrate that body weight can be lost merely by reducing the fat content of the diet without the need to voluntarily restrict food intake."

At the University of Alabama, doctors studied how dietary fat may help regulate the appetite. Both obese and nonobese volunteers were asked to eat to the point of feeling full while on diets that emphasized either low-fat, low-calorie foods (fruits, vegetables, grains, dried beans) or high-fat, high-calorie foods (meat, cheese). On the low-fat diet, people reported feeling full at 1,570 calories for the day; by comparison, it took 3,000 calories to produce feelings of fullness in the group on the high-fat diet. Those eating the high-fat meals consumed nearly twice as many calories each day—a fact that clearly influenced their body weight.

Researchers at the University of Illinois at Chicago and other institutions placed 18 women on a diet in which 37 percent of the calories came from fat. After four weeks, the women switched to a diet in which 20 percent of the calories came from fat, which they adhered to for an additional 20 weeks. Even though the women actually consumed more calories when eating the low-fat diet, they still lost weight, and significant amounts of it; body fat decreased 11.3 percent on the low-fat plan, while lean body weight increased 2.2 percent. On the high-fat diet, the women did not lose weight. Similar types of changes were seen in both obese and non-obese subjects.

Why does reducing your fat intake work so much better than counting calories? Cutting down on fat permits you to eat a wider variety and a greater volume of food than reducing your calorie consumption does. Also, for reasons that aren't well understood, cutting down on your fat intake seems to make it easier for you to override your internal weight regulator and thus to make permanent adjustments in your body weight.

Nutritional Advantages of Low-Fat Eating

A low-fat diet not only helps you control your weight, but offers other health benefits as well:

- **Lowers your cholesterol level.** Fats (particularly saturated fats*) are converted into cholesterol by your body and can cause your blood cholesterol levels to rise even more than dietary cholesterol does. Lowering the fat content of your diet helps you lower your blood cholesterol level and decrease your risk of developing heart disease.

- **Lowers your risk of cancer.** Studies show that diets that are very high in fat can increase the risk of certain cancers, particularly cancer of the colon and breast. High-fat diets also contribute to obesity, which increases a woman's risk of developing cancer of the uterus.

---

* *Saturated fats are recognized by the fact that they remain solid at room temperature (two examples of saturated fats are butter and shortening). Chemically, the difference between saturated and unsaturated fats is the number of hydrogen atoms they contain (saturated fats contain more than unsaturated fats).*

VEGETARIAN DIETS: NOT A LOW-FAT GUARANTEE

Many vegetarians assume—incorrectly—that a meat-free diet translates into a low-fat diet. After all, vegetables are generally low in fat, right? Right, but vegetarians do not live on vegetables alone. Although some very strict vegetarians avoid dairy products, most rely quite heavily on them as a source of protein, and this can cause problems with fat intake. For example, many vegetarians substitute cheese for meat, chicken, and fish, yet many cheeses derive more than 60 percent of their calories from fat (by comparison, skinless breast of chicken derives only 20 percent of its calories from fat, cod only 7 percent, and a lean cut of top sirloin beef only 28 percent).

Oils present another problem. Many vegetarian recipes call for lots of added fat in the form of oils, butter, or margarine. This extra fat is used to enhance the flavor of the low-fat vegetables, legumes, and grains that are the staples of many vegetarian dishes. Unfortunately, flavor is not the only thing added. Every tablespoon of oil adds 120 calories to the dish—100 percent of them fat calories.

And then there's the problem of snack foods and desserts. Cakes and cookies don't lose their fat when they're eaten by vegetarians.

So, if you're a vegetarian, don't assume you are automatically on a low-fat diet. Give as much thought to the percentage of fat in the foods you choose to eat as you do to the vitamins and minerals they contain, and you'll find it much easier to shed the extra pounds you need to lose.

Eat More and Lose Weight

Fat is dense in calories (which means that a lot of calories are packed into a small volume). In fact, fat is more than twice as dense in calories as carbohydrates (one gram of fat contains nine calories, while one gram of carbohydrates contains only four). So, by replacing high-fat foods in your diet with low-fat alternatives (including carbohydrates), you can eat a larger volume of food and still lose weight.

Here are a few examples of the difference in caloric density between some typical high-fat foods and some low-fat alternatives. The alternatives contain approximately the same number of calories, but look at how much more food you could eat.

One premium vanilla ice cream bar (370 calories, 66 percent from fat) or six frozen fruit bars (60 calories per bar, 0 percent from fat).

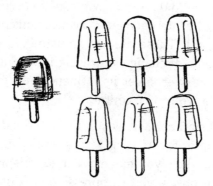

One-half cup of potato salad (340 calories, 58 percent from fat) or 3½ cups of fruit salad (90 calories per ½ cup serving, 0 percent from fat).

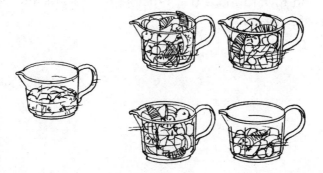

An ounce of mixed nuts (170 calories, 72 percent from fat) or a pound of carrots, beans, and broccoli (135 calories, 8 percent from fat).

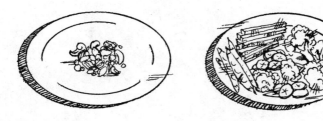

To lose weight comfortably—and, just as important, to keep it off—you need to decrease the amount of fat you eat. If you do that during the next 28 days, you will start to become more effective at overriding the internal regulatory mechanisms that are keeping you overweight. These dietary adjustments won't actually lower your set point, or change your weight regulator directly. But they will help you overpower its influence and gradually bring your weight under your own control.

This process will start as soon as you make these dietary changes, and it will continue for as long as you maintain them. What's more, unlike other diets you may have tried, this weight-loss plan won't become an obsessive or oppressive part of your life, preoccupying you throughout the day and draining your energy. Instead, it will involve some relatively painless shifts away from foods that increase your risk of obesity and your feelings of deprivation, and toward foods that promote weight loss and produce feelings of satisfaction.

6

INCREASING YOUR PHYSICAL ACTIVITY

Increasing the physical activity in your life is probably one of the most important changes you can make to ensure long-term weight loss and control of your weight regulator. Physical activity—not just exercise, but any kind of physical activity—increases the number of calories your body burns. Whether you do 20 minutes of gardening, take a five-minute walk, or go on a 40-minute run, when you are physically active your body burns more calories than it does when you're at rest.

Nevertheless, activity *by itself* is not the best technique for losing weight. Let's face it: You'd have to run nearly four miles or bike nearly ten to work off just one piece of chocolate cake with icing. You'd have to go nearly twice as far to work off a Big Mac and a small order of fries. Understandably, most folks would rather skip a meal than put in so much daily time and effort to lose weight.

So why do all weight-loss experts insist on including exercise in their programs—and why do we agree? The answer is simple:

People who increase their physical activity to lose weight are much more likely to keep the weight off. Those who don't exercise do very poorly over the long term. Studies show that 95 percent of all people who diet without making permanent changes in their lifestyles—including exercise—regain all the weight they lost. (Our own survey of TODAY show viewers in 1989 came up with a similar result.)

Why is exercise so effective at keeping weight off? Regular physical activity causes several changes in your body that have a positive impact on your weight-regulating system. Here's what physical activity does:

- It increases your metabolic rate—not only during exercise but for a period of time afterward.

- It helps to preserve lean muscle mass while reducing fat.

- It enhances self-image and an overall sense of well-being.

- It burns calories. (A half hour of brisk walking burns 200 calories, which may represent 10 to 15 percent of your total calories for the day.)

- It increases your ability to be attentive to your body, your needs, and the task of managing your eating.

- It may decrease appetite in obese people.

All this may sound fine on paper—of course, you want to override your weight regulator so you can maintain a lower weight. But what if you hate exercise? Or—as so many people claim—you simply can't find the time to fit an exercise program into your busy schedule? Are you doomed to stay overweight forever?

Not necessarily. You can find many other ways to increase your physical activity that will have the same ultimate weight-loss effect as exercise. Many people still believe that daily strenuous exercise is necessary to achieve and maintain significant weight loss. But research shows that any increase in daily activity—not just strenuous exercise—will burn calories, contribute to weight loss, and play an important role in keeping the weight off.

This means that you'll get the same weight-loss benefits whether you walk a mile or run it. It also means that simple activities related to your normal daily life will also contribute to weight loss— things like washing the car, making beds, and washing floors. The key is to increase your daily energy expenditure slowly but surely, whether through traditional exercise, routine physical activity, or—better yet—both.

In this chapter, we'll show you how to build other kinds of physical activity into your daily life. But we're not going to give up so easily on exercise. If, for just 28 days, you follow the exercise assignments built into our program, I predict you will turn into an exercise convert who not only enjoys exercise, but actually looks forward to doing it.

You can increase the benefits of exercise by involving yourself regularly in both aerobic activities and strength-training routines.

Aerobic Exercise

The body can utilize either glucose (from carbohydrates) or fat as a source of fuel for aerobic exercise. The proportion of each that is used depends, at least in part, on the intensity of the exercise. During low to moderate intensity exercise (such as brisk walking and jogging), the major source of fuel is fat. So, adding low intensity aerobic exercise to a weight-loss program enhances the loss of body fat. The powerful effect of exercise has been well demonstrated by research studies. In one study, for instance, a group of obese women were placed on a calorie-restricted diet. Half of the women were also started on a regular exercise regimen; the remaining women remained physically inactive. Among the women who exercised, 95 percent of their weight loss came from body fat. In the inactive group, only 64 percent of the weight loss came from fat; the rest was lost at the expense of muscles and other lean body tissues.

Strength Training

The effects of strength training are familiar to most of us. We've seen its miraculous effects on people at the gym, on the beach, and in the movies. But most overweight people are surprised to learn that strength training has an important role in weight loss. They mistakenly believe its benefits—building muscle—are reserved for thin people.

In fact, strength training can help you preserve muscle mass while losing weight. Several studies have shown that, even during periods of caloric restriction, strength training can not only preserve— but actually increase—muscle mass. Researchers at the University of Michigan proved this in two groups of women they studied. All of the women were placed on a calorie-restricted diet, but one group participated in a strength training program while the other half remained sedentary. While both groups of women lost weight overall, lean body weight increased in the women who were exercising (their muscle size and weight *increased*, so all of their weight loss was fat). Lean body weight *decreased* in the women who were sedentary, which means part of their overall weight loss resulted from the destruction of muscle tissue.

Increasing Your Commitment to Exercise

As you follow our program and become increasingly active in your day-to-day life, you may find that you actually want to devote more time to exercise than called for in our daily assignments. If so, I strongly recommend that you vary the activities you add. For example, I now jog three times a week, ride an indoor exercise bicycle twice a week, and ride a real bicycle outdoors once a week (on the seventh day, I sleep in). Varying my activities enables me to exercise different muscle groups and avoid boredom.

Activities you might want to combine in this way include walking or jogging, aerobics classes, exercise videotapes, hiking, tennis, running, swimming, and basketball. Be careful of the way commuting and other activities connected with exercise can eat up your time. Many people find that they spend as much time traveling to exercise (at a health club or track, for example), and then showering and dressing as they do on the exercise itself. Minimize travel by finding activities close to home or on your way to or from work.

To avoid having to shower and dress twice, do your exercise before you take your regular shower or at the end of the day.

The exercises you choose should give you a feeling of accomplishment and should fit your personality and lifestyle. Ask yourself a few questions to help determine an appropriate choice:

- Do you like being alone and out in the open, or does the busy, noisy atmosphere of a health club appeal to you more?

- Do you live in an area that makes long runs or walks especially appealing (and safe)?

- Do you live close to a high school track or a health club where it would be easier to work out?

- Are you someone who would prefer the contemplative pace of a long walk or the challenging intensity of a vigorous run?

Exercising When You Are Very Overweight

There is one benefit to being very overweight: The calorie-burning effect of exercise is magnified. For example, a 165-pound man who walks three miles will burn about 300 calories, while a 220-pound man will burn 390 calories walking the same distance. That's a bonus of 90 extra calories burned for carrying the extra 55 pounds that far.

The calorie-burning effect of exercise is magnified in heavier people because more work is required to move them the same distance (think about how much harder it is to walk a mile with a large pack on your back or a heavy baby in your arms than without that extra weight). So heavier people burn more calories than lighter people who are doing the same exercise. That's the good news.

The bad news is that people who are extremely overweight may have more problems with exercise than lighter people. They are more likely to have medical conditions that can influence their ability to exercise safely, such as diabetes or high blood pressure, and they are more prone to joint injuries if they jog or engage in other high impact activities. So, if you are very overweight—especially if you've also been very sedentary—be very careful about the way you increase your activity level. Start slowly and increase both the duration and intensity of your exercise gradually.

Give serious consideration to joining a class at your local "Y" or at a fitness facility that uses trained and certified instructors. If anyone tries to throw you into a high-intensity class in which you must struggle to keep up, walk (don't run) to the nearest exit and find another fitness program. Also, if you are significantly overweight, if you've been sedentary, or if you have any medical conditions that could be aggravated by exercise, consult with your physician before making any marked change in your level of physical activity. Your doctor will be able to advise you if any special precautions are needed in your particular case, and may be able to recommend a fitness program that is just right for your needs.

DIARY OF A REFORMED COUCH POTATO

(The Author's Personal Experience)

I'm married to a woman who exercises intensely every day (and who, by the way, has no problem maintaining a trim weight). Two years ago, when I decided to start my weight-regulating program, I tried running with her and fell hopelessly far behind. Instead of quitting, I took up walking. Then I gradually began building up my pace by jogging past one or two houses on each block of my route. For several months, I lengthened the jogging segments until I was able to run the entire three-mile route. Now I jog this route at least twice a week.

In 1995, at the urging of my children, I made another breakthrough in the exercise area: I started a strength-training routine. At first, my efforts were limited to a few simple exercises with five or ten pound dumbbells. Even with these simple routines, I felt a remarkable difference in muscle strength and tone almost immediately. Before long, I began a full-body routine on larger equipment with heavier weights and pulleys. Today, that equipment fills a former bedroom in our home, and you can find me working out on it every other day.

Since I started exercising, several changes occurred that have made exercise an increasingly important part of my life. I no longer think of exercise as punishment. Instead, I use my workouts as an opportunity for thinking time. I've also set up a system for rewarding myself for exercising. On the days I exercise, I give myself 30 minutes of free time before I start my day's work—time to call friends or to read the newspaper completely. I allow myself to go to work a little later on exercise days, and I don't feel guilty about it because I work more efficiently on these days.

As I gradually increased the level of physical activity in my life, I noticed that I began to feel better about myself. (I never felt bad about myself before; I just feel better now.) Although I started exercising for fitness—not to lose weight—I noticed that exercise also had some very positive effects on my attempts to lose weight. Exercise decreased my appetite and gave me the resolve to pass up high-calorie foods (after running three or four miles in the hills around my home, it's just not worth the small gratification I'd get eating that piece of cake). Exercise also has decreased the eating urges generated by my weight regulator. At the age of 59, I'm in the best shape of my life—and feeling better all the time.

To be honest, there is one thing exercise hasn't changed for me: I still have trouble getting started each day. When the alarm rings at 6 a.m., I can think of a million reasons to skip my run: The bed is warm. It's cold outside. I need more sleep. But I now know all these excuses are just my weight regulator's way of trying to get my weight back up to the level that it has set for me. Sounds crazy—but I am convinced it's true, and I won't let myself be tricked by my weight regulator's subconscious subterfuge. So—grudgingly—I roll out of bed, pull on my running shorts and head for the hills or my exercise bike.

The 28-day conditioning program outlined in this book will help you begin to make some of these same changes in your life. As you condition your body, you'll feel better about yourself. And, as you see the results of your efforts, you'll want to do more. Trust me. Even if you've never exercised before, don't rule it out until you've followed this program for 28 days. You'll be surprised how easy it is to make physical activity a part of your life.

7

MODIFYING YOUR EATING BEHAVIOR

Since the early 1960s, obesity researchers have been studying the eating patterns of overweight people to determine whether certain behaviors, such as eating rapidly or reading while eating, contribute to obesity. The initial studies suggested that some behaviors did in fact play a role in obesity. The researchers concluded that people who changed their behavior would be more successful at losing weight and keeping it off. Since then, most weight-loss programs have used some elements of behavior modification (or behavior therapy, as it is often called) in the design of their recommended activities.

Most obesity experts now believe that making behavioral therapy part of a weight-loss program increases the likelihood that the weight lost will be kept off after the program is concluded. However, experience shows that some individuals benefit much more from behavior modification than others do. Since it's hard to predict who will get the best results from behavior therapy, I strongly urge you to try as many behavioral techniques as you can, continuing to use the ones that work well for you, and discarding the rest.

Let's take a look at the main categories of behavior modification methods and the techniques in each of these areas:

Stimulus control. With this technique, you will attempt to reduce the external factors that might trigger you to eat. Studies show that some people are much more likely to eat—even when they don't want to—if they are exposed to the sight or smell of food. Thus, you need to reduce the temptations that can lead to inappropriate eating, particularly at times other than predetermined mealtimes.

To decrease the frequency and intensity of these exposures to food, you can try adopting behaviors such as:

- Shop only with a detailed shopping list and on a full stomach, to prevent impulse buying.

- Keep food—except for fruits and vegetables—stored away in opaque containers and out of sight, so you will not think about eating them every time you walk by. (Most fruits and vegetables, of course, are healthful, nonfat foods that you can eat whenever you feel like having a snack.)

- Use smaller plates to make portions appear larger than they actually are.

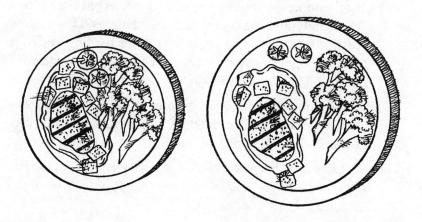

- When sitting down to a meal, don't leave serving bowls on the table. They make it very hard to resist the temptation to have seconds. Before you sit down at the dinner table, place excess food in storage containers and put them in the refrigerator.

- Whenever possible, do all your eating in one place in your home, preferably in a dining room that is separate from the kitchen.

- Remove all food from the table as soon as you have finished eating; put leftovers in those opaque containers and keep them out of view.

Self-monitoring. With this technique, you will observe—and record in detail—everything related to your eating. This may involve keeping a diary or a log in which you note everything you eat and the circumstances surrounding your eating. For example, you might record information such as: What time did I eat? How much did I eat? Where did I eat? Why did I eat? What was I feeling at the time? How did I feel afterward? With information such as this, you can begin to make changes more conducive to weight loss, and monitor your success in adopting these behavioral transformations.

Here are some other self-monitoring strategies:

- Review and evaluate your accomplishments at the end of every day.

- Concentrate on your eating so you can record the process accurately and make appropriate changes. Don't allow distractions like watching television or reading to divert your thoughts away from eating. Paying attention to your food will help you find more pleasure in it—and eat less.

- Slow your eating. Monitor yourself as you chew more slowly; put your fork down between bites; allow 30 seconds to elapse between bites.

- Let five minutes pass before you get up and go for second portions. (You'll probably decide that you don't want the second helping after all.)

- Review your written record at regular intervals (at least weekly) to identify problems that need to be solved and to recognize successful strategies that could be used more often.

Cognitive change. Many people who are overweight feel negatively about themselves, or are so sensitive to negative comments of others, that they sabotage their own weight-loss attempts. Behavioral therapy tries to change those negative beliefs, attitudes and responses, and alter the way people perceive their efforts at losing weight. You might be helped along in this process by individual or group therapy, which can help change your self-image and the way you respond to the world around you.

To promote cognitive change:

- Do not measure your self-worth on a bathroom scale.

- Use a relaxation technique to calm your mind and body before you eat anything.

- Try to distinguish between physiological hunger and cravings that have an emotional cause.

- Make sure your short- and long-term weight-loss goals are realistic.

- Plan to lose weight very gradually, over a long period of time.

- Do not let yourself believe that a slip in your program means you're a failure. Restart your weight-loss program as soon as you can.

Reinforcement. Usually, losing weight is, in and of itself, a rewarding experience for someone who is overweight. The process of reinforcement involves making deliberate attempts to further enhance the positive side of the weight-loss experience by creating additional rewards.

Here are some examples of reinforcement:

- Enlist support and encouragement from your loved ones and friends.

- Reward yourself for sticking with the plan, not just for the weight loss you've achieved. The rewards do not have to be expensive, but they should be personally meaningful.

- Look at your new body in the mirror, and let yourself enjoy the image reflecting back at you.

8

SELF-MONITORING
AND RECORDING
YOUR PROGRESS

You have now learned three of the major strategies you need to use to override your internal weight regulator. You've learned how to reduce the fat content of your diet, how to become more physically active, and what changes to make in your eating behavior. A fourth important strategy involves self-monitoring and keeping records of your accomplishments. Putting this strategy into action is crucial to your weight-loss success.

Most people assume that weighing themselves is all the monitoring they need to do. But you must do more if you want to know which parts of your weight-loss program are working for you, and which are not. Careful monitoring and recording of your activities will reveal what you're doing right and which areas you need to improve.

Active self-monitoring and recording are very effective tools for making lasting changes. They compel you to take possession of your own behavior, because they enable you to identify problem areas that require your attention and work.

Alternatives for Monitoring

There are many different systems for monitoring and recording your progress, and you've probably encountered some of them in diets you've tried in the past. These systems include everything from complex wall posters to extremely detailed diaries that document every morsel of food you eat and every mood you experience during the day.

Some dieters have found these elaborate food diaries to be valuable, and if you're one of those people, I don't want to discourage you from keeping one now. People have told me that keeping a diary helps them greatly in understanding why, and under what circumstances, they overeat. The diary enables them to record the social situations that may trigger them to overeat, and to identify the people, settings, moods, and feelings that cause them to reach for food even after they've already eaten enough to satisfy their hunger. In keeping track of everything they eat and what they are feeling when they eat, they may discover, for example, that they use food to feel better when they are angry, anxious, or lonely.

For many individuals, however, detailed food diaries are simply too much work and trouble, incompatible with their busy lifestyles. One tongue-in-cheek theory is that people who lose weight on a program built around a food diary do so because all the record-keeping leaves them with no time to eat!

The monitoring and recording system I'll ask you to follow for the next 28 days is much simpler. It is an uncomplicated approach that forces you to think about what you're doing, bringing the strategies in this program into conscious awareness. I've narrowed down the monitoring parameters to just three key elements of this program:

1. The amount of fat you're consuming

2. The amount of physical activity in your day

3. The way you are eating your food

Each day, it will take just two to three minutes to evaluate how you've done in these three areas, and to translate that evaluation into a visual representation of your progress.

The Basics of the Monitoring System

Here is how the self-monitoring program in this book works. You will spend two to three minutes at the end of each day reflecting upon your accomplishments by asking yourself these questions:

- Was I successful in reducing the amount of dietary fat I consumed today? Did I avoid foods with more than 30 percent fat content and increase my intake of foods that get less than 30 percent of their calories from fat?

- Did I complete the exercise assignment for the day (or an equivalent physical activity that I designed for myself)?

- Did I succeed in changing my eating behaviors—specifically, slowing my eating pace and consistently taking 30 seconds between bites? Am I paying attention to how and what I eat? Am I leaving the table once I am no longer hungry?

As you respond to these questions over the next 28 days (and in the weeks and months thereafter), you'll use one of the simple Self-Monitoring tearout charts that appear in this book to record your answers. At the end of each day, take a moment to evaluate yourself and record your day's accomplishments on the chart. As shown in the key, use a pencil or pen to fill in the entire circle if you fully accomplished a particular goal. Fill in just half the circle if you accomplished only part of that goal. And if you had a bad day with respect to that component of the program, leave the circle empty.

So, for example, at day's end you will ask yourself how well you fared in minimizing the fat content of your diet. If you ate no foods containing more than 30 percent fat (or very few of those foods in very small portions), and you ate many foods with less than 10 percent fat, fill in the entire fat circle for the day. At the other extreme, if you went off the plan totally, leave the circle completely blank. And if you ended up somewhere in-between—perhaps doing well for three meals, but blowing it with a high-fat snack late at night . . . or topping a salad with cold cuts and high-fat dressing—color in one-half of the "Cut Fat" circle. Don't worry about being exactly accurate with this scoring system. Your approximations will be enough to reveal what's working for you, and where your problems lie.

SELF–MONITORING CHART

	MONDAY	TUESDAY	WEDNESDAY	THURSDAY	FRIDAY	SATURDAY	SUNDAY
Cut Fat	○	○	○	○	○	○	○
Increase Exercise	○	○	○	○	○	○	○
Modify Behavior	○	○	○	○	○	○	○

	MONDAY	TUESDAY	WEDNESDAY	THURSDAY	FRIDAY	SATURDAY	SUNDAY
Cut Fat	○	○	○	○	○	○	○
Increase Exercise	○	○	○	○	○	○	○
Modify Behavior	○	○	○	○	○	○	○

met goal ●   partially met goal ◐   missed goal ○

Each day, perform the same scoring ritual with physical activity. If you complete your exercise assignment for the day (or an equivalent activity), fill in the whole circle. If not, either fill in half the circle or leave it completely blank.

Score yourself behaviorally, too. Are you pacing yourself at every meal? Are you paying attention to what you're eating? Are you leaving the table when you're no longer hungry? If you answer yes to these questions, fill in the entire circle for that day. If you can't be quite so affirmative in your responses, fill in whatever area seems appropriate.

Keep in mind that you will be making general, qualitative evaluations of how you're doing. You don't need to calculate how many fat grams you've consumed that day, nor will you be adding up calories. Instead, try to reach fair and realistic judgments of how well you're doing, and then record those evaluations on the chart.

Each day, as you are filling in the circles that chart your progress, ask yourself not just "What did I do today?" but also "Why?" If, in fact, you left a circle blank because you had a high-fat day, try to learn why you didn't do better. Did you give in to the temptation of the sweet rolls or doughnuts provided at a breakfast meeting? Did you snack on fatty foods while preparing dinner? Did you indulge in a hefty helping of ice cream because you were feeling bored or upset? As you answer the question why, you will begin to recognize the specific problems that undermine your weight-loss efforts. Then you can make adjustments in your daily routine that will help you deal effectively with those issues.

The Big Picture

Each day, after you record your scores for fat intake, eating behavior, and exercise, enter this information immediately on one of the Self-Monitoring tearout charts in this book. This chart should be placed on your refrigerator door, on a bulletin board in the kitchen, or in some other conspicuous place in your home or office where you will see it frequently. As you fill in the circles, one day after another, you'll see patterns emerge that reveal your problem areas.

Filling in the chart—and more specifically, analyzing it—will enable you to learn what helps and hinders you and to put that knowledge into future plans and action.

My own recent history illustrates the value of this process. I thought I was doing a pretty good job of maintaining a regular exercise program—until I actually started monitoring and charting my physical activity. That's when the true patterns emerged. My chart revealed that I was barely getting in two days of exercise a week, and that weekdays were my most difficult time. I also could see that travel days were a real problem; I rarely exercised when I was on the road.

Once I became aware of my actual exercise patterns, I changed the way I scheduled my weekdays, making exercise a much more important priority. By making it the first "appointment" on my schedule instead of the last, I increased the number of sessions to six per week. I removed the obstacles that kept me from exercising when I traveled by calling ahead to hotels, and making reservations only in those that had exercise rooms. Incidentally, when I travel, I continue to monitor and record this information on a pocket calendar, transferring these data to the chart as soon as I return home.

The chart, then, is a visual portrait of your eating, exercising, and behavior patterns. At a glance, it can reveal how you're doing, and identify where you need to begin concentrating more attention. It not only will help you identify weak areas, but—if displayed in the right location—can also be highly motivating. I keep my chart on a door in my office, where I (and everyone else in the office) can look at it frequently. (If you'd rather keep your chart private, post it in a place where everyone who walks by won't see it.)

Each time you examine your chart during the next 28 days, see whether you can detect patterns that are creating problems for you. If many empty or half-empty circles appear during a particular week, or if they appear repeatedly on a particular day of the week, ask yourself, "Why?" The answer to that simple question may help you pinpoint particular situations or emotions that are triggering problems.

Let's look at some common patterns and areas of difficulty that people have noticed when using these or similar charts. With each case study, you'll be able to identify a problem pattern, and you'll see how recognizing that pattern made it easier to determine the changes that were necessary.

PATTERN I: TRAVEL TROUBLE

A businesswoman named Barbara travels two to three days a week as part of her job. Barbara is typically on the road every Tuesday through Thursday, with meetings filling up her very long days. She stays overnight in hotels two nights a week. In the past, she rarely exercised during those out-of-town trips, and she ate a higher-fat diet than she did when she was home.

Barbara understands why she had trouble on those travel days. "The time zone shifts are hard on me," she says. "It's difficult for me to think about exercising at 7 a.m. in New York when my brain is still functioning on Los Angeles time, where it's only 4 a.m. And in the evening when I get back to my hotel, I'm hesitant to take walks by myself at night in strange cities and neighborhoods."

When traveling, Barbara says she sometimes had no time to eat breakfast or lunch, except perhaps for a quick visit to a fast-food

SELF-MONITORING CHART — BARBARA'S WEEK 1&2

	MONDAY	TUESDAY	WEDNESDAY	THURSDAY	FRIDAY	SATURDAY	SUNDAY
Cut Fat	met goal	partially met goal	missed goal	missed goal	met goal	met goal	met goal
Increase Exercise	met goal	missed goal	missed goal	missed goal	met goal	met goal	met goal
Modify Behavior	met goal	missed goal	missed goal	missed goal	partially met goal	met goal	met goal

	MONDAY	TUESDAY	WEDNESDAY	THURSDAY	FRIDAY	SATURDAY	SUNDAY
Cut Fat	met goal	missed goal	partially met goal	missed goal	met goal	met goal	met goal
Increase Exercise	met goal	missed goal	met goal	missed goal	met goal	met goal	met goal
Modify Behavior	met goal	missed goal	partially met goal	missed goal	partially met goal	partially met goal	met goal

met goal ●   partially met goal ◗   missed goal ○

restaurant. And on long airplane flights, even her best efforts at eating wisely ran into obstacles. "Too often, the flight attendants told me they were out of the fruit plate, but I could have all the lasagna or greasy chicken I wanted!"

As you can see in Barbara's chart, Tuesdays through Thursdays were her only problem days. She eventually learned to overcome her stumbling blocks on those days. Barbara now books rooms only in hotels that have (or have access to) indoor exercise facilities. She calls ahead to be sure the health club is open in the evening when she has time to use it, and she asks whether the facility has enough equipment to go around if several hotel guests show up at the same time.

Barbara now relies on hotel room service for her breakfasts and late-night dinners, carefully choosing low-fat items from the menu. When she flies, she calls ahead to the airline and requests a special meal. A low-fat or vegetarian plate is always waiting for her. Before boarding the plane for long flights, she buys a cup of nonfat yogurt in the airport, and carries it on board. This makes it much easier to refuse the high-fat peanuts that are offered with soft drinks after takeoff. The yogurt also keeps Barbara more comfortable when she's the last one served on a jam-packed widebody.

PATTERN 2: CARPOOL CRUNCH

An accountant named Marilyn drives the morning carpool to her child's school on Mondays and Wednesdays. The 35-minute round trip consumes the time that she would otherwise use for exercise.

"On the other mornings of the week, I put an exercise video in the VCR as soon as my daughter is out the door, and I work out for half an hour," said Marilyn. "But on carpool days, I have no time for physical activity."

As you can see in Marilyn's chart, carpool days became days that she didn't exercise, and over time, her conscientious weight-loss efforts the rest of the week were undermined.

Marilyn finally took back control, however. She now sets her alarm clock earlier on the days she drives the carpool. "Two mornings a week, the exercise video goes into the VCR at 6 a.m.," she says. "At first, I wasn't excited at the prospect of starting those days so early. But the exercise itself is invigorating, even at that early hour—and I've begun to see that it helps keep me on track with the rest of my weight-control program."

SELF–MONITORING CHART				MARILYN'S WEEK	1&2	
	MONDAY	TUESDAY	WEDNESDAY	THURSDAY	FRIDAY	SATURDAY	SUNDAY
Cut Fat	●	●	●	●	●	●	●
Increase Exercise	○	●	○	●	●	●	●
Modify Behavior	●	◑	◑	○	●	◑	●

	MONDAY	TUESDAY	WEDNESDAY	THURSDAY	FRIDAY	SATURDAY	SUNDAY
Cut Fat	◑	◑	●	●	●	●	●
Increase Exercise	○	●	○	●	●	●	○
Modify Behavior	◑	◑	●	●	●	●	●

met goal ●　　　partially met goal ◑　　　missed goal ○

PATTERN 3: WEEKEND WEAKNESS

Larry lost 25 pounds over the past year, but his success stalled very early on. As his chart shows, Larry did extremely well on weekdays in all three key areas—low-fat dining, eating behavior, and exercise. "My weekdays are very structured, and I can make time for everything," he said. "But the weekends are a really difficult time for me. I enjoy sleeping in, my two kids have their Little League and soccer games at varying times, and there are social events where I have no control over the food that is being served. I simply fall apart on Saturdays and Sundays."

When these patterns became clear to him—and when he realized how they were interfering with his weight-loss efforts—Larry took action. Now, every Friday night, he plans the upcoming weekend as carefully as he plans his workdays. He schedules "appointments" for exercise, making physical activity a top priority. He's waking up much earlier now on Saturdays and Sundays, but he also allows himself the luxury of a catnap during the day. At social gatherings, Larry pays attention to what he eats and paces himself during meals, even though the result is often that he's the last at the table to finish. Since making these changes, Larry has steadily lost weight, with no backsliding on the weekends.

SELF–MONITORING CHART				LARRY'S WEEK 1&2		
	MONDAY	TUESDAY	WEDNESDAY	THURSDAY	FRIDAY	SATURDAY	SUNDAY
Cut Fat	●	●	●	●	●	○	◑
Increase Exercise	●	●	○	◑	●	○	○
Modify Behavior	●	●	●	●	●	○	○

	MONDAY	TUESDAY	WEDNESDAY	THURSDAY	FRIDAY	SATURDAY	SUNDAY
Cut Fat	●	●	●	●	●	◑	○
Increase Exercise	●	●	●	●	●	○	○
Modify Behavior	◑	◑	●	●	●	○	○

met goal ●   partially met goal ◑   missed goal ○

PATTERN 4: WEEKDAY WOES

Josephine's problems were precisely the opposite of Larry's. She did extremely well on weekends when the days were much more her own, and when she had enough time to exercise and prepare low-fat meals. But during the week, the pressures and stresses of working full-time and keeping her household running smoothly left her eating on the run and skipping her exercise sessions.

SELF–MONITORING CHART				JOSEPHINE'S WEEK	1&2	
	MONDAY	TUESDAY	WEDNESDAY	THURSDAY	FRIDAY	SATURDAY	SUNDAY
Cut Fat	○	○	○	◐	○	●	●
Increase Exercise	○	●	○	○	○	●	●
Modify Behavior	○	○	○	○	○	●	●

	MONDAY	TUESDAY	WEDNESDAY	THURSDAY	FRIDAY	SATURDAY	SUNDAY
Cut Fat	○	○	○	○	◐	●	●
Increase Exercise	●	○	○	○	○	●	●
Modify Behavior	○	○	○	○	◐	◐	●

met goal ●   partially met goal ◐   missed goal ○

"My chart showed what I should've known all along, but didn't," says Josephine. "I wasn't doing well during the week. And that made even my best dieting efforts on the weekends relatively unproductive."

Josephine finally decided to alter her lifestyle. Instead of large lunches in the cafeteria with her coworkers, she now brown-bags it with a low-fat lunch from home. The simpler meal leaves her ample time for a 30-minute walk during her lunch hour, and some of her friends at work are now walking with her. With these simple changes, she has gotten on track and is continuing to lose a little more weight each week.

Some people discover that their difficulties seem to be concentrated in only one of the rows on the chart. Here again, some clear patterns often develop. Let's look at a few examples of the most common ones.

PATTERN 5: FATTY FOOD FOUL-UPS

Bruce began his weight-loss program with a strong commitment to succeed. From the beginning, he started exercising and eating slowly, and his chart reflected those successes. But he had a lot of empty circles on the line that represented his efforts to reduce dietary fat.

"I hate to pass the buck," says Bruce, "but my wife was completely unsupportive of my program from the first day onward. I married someone who was born lucky: She has a naturally high metabolism. She has always been thin, and she doesn't feel she has to make any personal sacrifices to help me stick with this program. When she shops, she buys lots of high-fat foods, because that's what she likes. When she cooks, she cooks high-fat dishes. And when I come home from work in the evening, she has dinner—a high-fat dinner—waiting on the table for us."

Bruce finally realized that it was up to him to take control of this problem. Even though it initially seemed odd to do so, Bruce now shops for most of his own food, and his wife shops for hers. On weekends, he prepares some of his dinners for the following week and freezes or refrigerates them, using the microwave oven to heat them up throughout the week.

"It's not the ideal situation," says Bruce. "But it works without driving a wedge between me and my wife. And I'm finally filling in the circles on the fat reduction row of my chart."

SELF–MONITORING CHART — BRUCE'S WEEK 1&2

	MONDAY	TUESDAY	WEDNESDAY	THURDAY	FRIDAY	SATURDAY	SUNDAY
Cut Fat	○	○	◑	○	○	○	○
Increase Exercise	●	○	●	●	◑	●	●
Modify Behavior	●	●	●	●	○	◑	●

	MONDAY	TUESDAY	WEDNESDAY	THURDAY	FRIDAY	SATURDAY	SUNDAY
Cut Fat	○	○	○	○	○	○	◑
Increase Exercise	●	●	○	●	●	●	●
Modify Behavior	●	◑	●	●	◑	●	◑

met goal ●   partially met goal ◑   missed goal ○

PATTERN 6: FROM EXERCISE TO EXHAUSTION

Lydia was on the track team in high school, and although it's been more than 20 years since her last competitive race, she still feels as though she has to go for the gold whenever she laces up her jogging shoes.

"It was so hard to find time to exercise, and my chart showed that," she says. "So when I did jog, which was usually only on weekends, I really pushed myself. I ran as far and as hard as I could, figuring I could make up for the days I missed. But I often paid the price with pulled muscles, sore knees, or blisters. Those aches and pains would force me to stay away from exercise for a week or two at a time."

Rather than pushing herself to the limit every week or two, Lydia would be far better off walking just a few blocks every day. And that's exactly what she finally decided to do.

SELF–MONITORING CHART				LYDIA'S WEEK	1&2	
	MONDAY	TUESDAY	WEDNESDAY	THURSDAY	FRIDAY	SATURDAY	SUNDAY
Cut Fat	◑	●	●	●	◑	●	◑
Increase Exercise	○	○	○	○	○	○	●
Modify Behavior	●	○	◑	●	○	●	◑

	MONDAY	TUESDAY	WEDNESDAY	THURSDAY	FRIDAY	SATURDAY	SUNDAY
Cut Fat	◑	●	●	◑	●	◑	●
Increase Exercise	●	○	○	○	○	●	○
Modify Behavior	◑	●	●	●	●	○	●

met goal ● partially met goal ◑ missed goal ○

"Every morning, I leave for work 15 minutes earlier than I used to, and I park in a lot about a mile from my office," she says. "I walk several blocks to work, and then walk back in the late afternoon when I go back to my car. I also try to add an additional mile at lunch. Of course, to me, these short walks don't seem like real exercise. But I feel great. I've never suffered an injury this way, and I'm now filling in the exercise row on my chart five days a week."

PATTERN 7: FEEDING FRENZY

Mel always seemed to be rushing through the day. He raced out the door every morning on his way to work. His day was jammed with appointments. And even at night, he attended meetings of committees on which he had volunteered to serve. So when he started this weight-loss program, you could have predicted that he would have trouble slowing down his eating pace.

"I did very well shifting to low-fat foods, and three mornings a week, I woke up early to go to the gym," says Mel. "But I always ate staring at the clock. I'd eat breakfast on my feet. I'd sometimes eat dinner in the car while driving to meetings. Not only didn't I pause 30 seconds between bites—it felt like I ate entire meals in not much more than 30 seconds!"

SELF–MONITORING CHART						MEL'S WEEK	1&2
	MONDAY	TUESDAY	WEDNESDAY	THURSDAY	FRIDAY	SATURDAY	SUNDAY
Cut Fat	●	●	●	●	●	●	●
Increase Exercise	●	○	●	○	●	○	○
Modify Behavior	○	○	○	○	○	○	○

	MONDAY	TUESDAY	WEDNESDAY	THURSDAY	FRIDAY	SATURDAY	SUNDAY
Cut Fat	◑	●	●	●	●	◑	●
Increase Exercise	●	○	●	○	●	●	○
Modify Behavior	○	○	○	○	○	◑	◑

met goal ●   partially met goal ◑   missed goal ○

Mel finally recognized that to succeed in this program, he would have to give himself more time for meals. He made adjustments in his work schedule so he wasn't due at his desk until 8:30 a.m. (instead of 8). That allowed him a more leisurely pace in the morning—and a chance for a breakfast that he could eat slowly. He used a similar strategy at lunch and dinnertime, too.

"I just decided that losing weight was a priority," says Mel. "And that meant giving myself a few things, like a full half-hour for lunch each day. It also meant resigning from some committees so dinners could be more relaxed." As Mel has filled in more circles in the eating behavior portion of his chart, his weight has gradually declined.

PATTERN 8: COPING WITH CHAOS

Nothing seemed to be going right for Karen. She had tried a dozen or more diets in the past, and ultimately failed on all of them. With the program in this book, things didn't start off much better.

SELF-MONITORING CHART						KAREN'S WEEK 1&2	
	MONDAY	TUESDAY	WEDNESDAY	THURSDAY	FRIDAY	SATURDAY	SUNDAY
Cut Fat	○	○	◑	○	○	◑	◑
Increase Exercise	◑	○	○	○	●	○	○
Modify Behavior	○	○	○	○	○	○	○
	MONDAY	TUESDAY	WEDNESDAY	THURSDAY	FRIDAY	SATURDAY	SUNDAY
Cut Fat	○	●	◑	○	◑	●	○
Increase Exercise	○	○	○	○	○	○	○
Modify Behavior	○	○	○	○	○	○	○

met goal ●   partially met goal ◑   missed goal ○

"I'd look at my chart, and I was having problems in every area," says Karen. "Particularly in the first couple of weeks, there were hardly any filled-in circles. It was so frustrating."

Karen was forced to do some soul-searching. She analyzed both her chart and her lifestyle, and concluded that she was trying to do too much. As a result, she wasn't really getting anything done.

I advised Karen to start again, but this time to take small steps, targeting one area of the program at a time. For two weeks, she worked exclusively on cutting back the fat content of her diet. Once she felt she had gained control in that area, she moved on to eating behavior, concentrating on eating those low-fat foods more slowly. Then, two weeks later, she began to exercise, too.

"It took more than the first 28 days for me to get all the elements of the program working," says Karen. "But I'm so glad I stuck with it. I'm not only losing weight, but I feel a tremendous sense of accomplishment."

The Power of Self-Monitoring

By reviewing your own chart and analyzing your entries, you too can spot problems quickly and make whatever changes are necessary to keep yourself on the road to weight loss. At least once a week, take the time to look at the patterns of circles on the chart. Continually evaluating how you're doing will allow you to identify problems and correct them before they become ingrained habits.

Your ultimate goal, of course, is to completely fill in all the circles on the chart. When you can do that, you are assured of losing weight. When circles are empty, the chart should help you understand why, and motivate you to make some changes.

Every problem you uncover really does have a solution—if you are seriously committed to losing weight. For instance, during the cold and rainy days of winter, or the hot and humid days of summer, you may be tempted to skip exercising because the weather outdoors makes it uncomfortable. But a trip to the health club or the use of an exercise video at home can keep the elements from interfering with your weight-loss efforts. So can a visit to the local shopping mall, where you can walk to your heart's content under cover. (Go to the mall early in the day when the corridors are uncrowded; many malls, in fact, have organized walking groups that plan walks before the mall stores open.)

Self-monitoring is not just about finding your weaknesses and problem areas. It is just as useful for highlighting your strengths in this program. As you look closely at days when you've done very well, ask yourself what you can learn from those experiences. How can you apply the strategies that brought you success in those situations to other areas in which you still might be having problems?

Remember, self-monitoring is a dynamic process. Filling in the circles is just the first step. You need to feed this information back into the program, and use it to gradually increase your control over your eating choices and your exercise patterns.

Moving Ahead

One final point deserves emphasis. The charts and records are not valuable in themselves; it's all in how you use them. As you begin this conditioning program, view each day's self-monitoring and charting as a springboard for the next day's efforts. While you evaluate your progress, you also refocus your energies and get a fast start on the following day. Charting is a learning tool; use it to determine what you need to do to override the upward pressure of your weight regulator.

PART III
TAKING IT OFF,
KEEPING IT OFF:
THE PROGRAM

9

THE ULTIMATE GOAL: FITNESS

If you are anything like the average person who buys this book, you have just one goal in mind: weight loss. This book will help you realize that goal, but it can take you far beyond that if you follow all aspects of our program in a consistent manner. It can help you achieve a new level of fitness that will truly change your life forever.

What do I mean by "fitness"? I'm talking about: getting up in the morning and really looking forward to the day; reaching the end of the day without feeling exhausted; exercising and enjoying it; lowering your blood pressure and cholesterol levels, and reducing your risk of heart disease, stroke and cancer; and feeling younger and more vigorous than you have in years.

Weight loss alone cannot do these things for you—especially when it is solely accomplished through severe caloric restriction. The diet that forces you to eat nothing but fruit for days on end, that denies you any significant source of protein, that refuses you solid foods—all in the name of weight loss—cannot lead you to lifelong fitness. Indeed, the weight loss such diets produce is likely to be short-lived.

We have taken a different approach in this program, because we believe that weight loss alone is not an appropriate goal. While some of the health benefits you will derive from this program will be directly related to losing weight, many of them—perhaps some of the most important—will not be related to the weight loss itself. They will come instead as a result of the lifestyle changes you'll be making in the weeks and months ahead, like reducing your fat intake and increasing your activity level.

The Benefits of Lifestyle Change

Reducing your fat intake will not only cause you to lose weight, but also help lower your cholesterol level and decrease your risk of developing heart disease. Cutting back on the amount of fat you eat can even help lower your risk of developing some cancers (particularly colon and breast).

Increasing your activity level as called for in our program will not only promote weight loss, but also raise your energy level, enhance your endurance, increase your muscle tone, and improve your strength. You can't achieve these results with crash diets. Regular exercise offers several other health benefits: It decreases your risk of heart disease and stroke; it reduces your risk of developing high blood pressure, osteoporosis and certain types of cancers; and it increases your life expectancy (in one recent study, researchers found that men who exercised regularly and improved their level of fitness were 44 percent less likely to die during a five-year period than men who were inactive).

The exercise assignments you'll be doing will also improve the way you feel generally. Exercise helps relieve stress and triggers the release of endorphins, chemicals that have a natural mood-elevating and pain-relieving effect. Just ask people who exercise regularly—they don't do it just for the physical effects, or even for the weight-loss benefits.

I don't mean to underplay the importance of losing weight, which offers many benefits in and of itself. Losing weight can help bring high blood pressure under control and can help lower elevated cholesterol and triglyceride levels. For people taking blood pressure drugs or cholesterol-lowering medications, this can result in lower doses or, in some cases, even stopping the medicines altogether. Taking off excess weight can also help people with diabetes bring their disease under control and minimize their risk of complications.

But let's stop thinking just about weight loss. As you progress through our program, focus instead on your overall good health. And, as you face each day's assignments, think of it as "taking care of yourself." If you do take care of yourself, the weight loss will take care of itself.

Keys to Success

Over the years, I've talked to many people who lost large amounts of weight and kept it off for long periods of time—5, 10, 20 years, or more. The 28-day plan you are about to start is based on the successful strategies they used to achieve their goals. Here's why these people have done so well for so long.

- **They have a concrete plan for losing weight and keeping it off, and they continue to follow it.** Their eating and exercise efforts have a well-defined structure. These people are guided by rules, and even when they have lost their weight and are able to relax a little, they remain committed to the principles and the plan that got them to their goal.

- **They are patient, and they are willing to accept progress that comes slowly.** They do not require immediate gratification, and they do not become discouraged with slow progress. They accept weight plateaus as normal.

- **They pay *active* attention to their eating.** They elevate eating to a conscious level, paying active attention to such things as the appearance, taste, smell, and consistency of their food. With food still on the plate, these people make a deliberate decision about whether to stop eating or to continue.

- **They eat a diet that is low in fat, but varied and interesting.** They eat a broad variety of foods, and they experiment frequently with new foods. They view themselves as making better food choices rather than dieting.

- **They engage in regular physical activity.** They set aside regular times for exercise on a near-daily basis. They are more concerned with the regularity of their exercise sessions than with the intensity of their routines. These people increase the intensity and duration of their exercise very gradually. They vary their activities and their exercise locations, and often exercise with others.

- **They do not eat food to relieve feelings of stress.** They are aware of the effects that stress has on their lives (and on their eating), and they have developed effective alternative strategies for dealing with stress. They use relaxation techniques or exercise to relieve tension, instead of eating.

- **They monitor their eating behaviors and physical activities on a regular basis.** They keep exercise logs and food diaries, and they weigh themselves regularly (but not more than once a day). Every day, they spend a moment or two reflecting on the day's weight management activities.

- **They recover quickly when they have a lapse.** They don't wait until the next week or the next month to get back on track—they don't even wait until tomorrow. They start the work of recovering immediately.

- **They feel supported by family and friends.** These people ask for support from those around them, and usually receive it. They share progress (and setbacks) with family, friends, and coworkers without fear of criticism.

- **They believe in and care about themselves.** These people felt good about themselves before they lost weight, and they feel good about themselves now. When overweight, they ignored disparaging remarks by others. Now that they have lost weight, they do not take others' congratulatory remarks too seriously. They lost weight for health reasons or to feel more comfortable, not to please others. These people are unwilling to jeopardize their health by fasting or using fad diets in order to lose weight.

In the 28-day Conditioning Phase that follows, you'll learn the strategies that will help you adopt these ten keys and make your weight loss long-term.

The Program Design

The program is divided into three parts: a 28-day Conditioning Phase, a Continuity Phase, and a Maintenance Phase. Although all phases are based on the same scientific principles, each one is specifically designed to deal with the different issues that come up over time. You will find more detailed descriptions of each phase in the next three chapters, along with detailed instructions on what you need to do.

The 28-day Conditioning Phase (Chapter 10) is a highly structured plan designed to change the way you react to food and exercise, and to teach you new techniques for weight management. Each day, you will find specific assignments related to your fat intake, your eating behaviors, and your activity level. It is important that you follow these assignments as closely as possible, and that you complete the chart that is provided for each day. This will help to keep your initial weight loss in a safe, but satisfying range, while promoting a steady increase in your fitness level. Every day, you will also find new information and new techniques you can use to enhance your weight-loss efforts.

The Continuity Phase (Chapter 11) is designed for people who still have more weight to lose after the Conditioning Phase is completed (yes, there are some fortunate people who will reach their final goals in just 28 days). This phase is much less structured, although you will still be asked to continue your newly learned eating, exercise, and monitoring behaviors. During this phase, however, the responsibility for selecting specific assignments will be yours. You will have an opportunity at this time to customize the program to meet your particular likes and dislikes. Chapter 11 contains a ten-week plan that you can tailor to your needs, but its open-ended design will enable you to continue to use those strategies that have worked for you in the past 28 days, and to adopt new ones that can keep you on track to lose all the weight you want to lose.

Finally, once you reach your weight-loss goal, you'll begin the Maintenance Phase (Chapter 12). In this part of the program, your aim is to keep off the weight you've already lost. The most difficult part of any weight-loss plan is to maintain your success over the long term, but you'll learn strategies for helping you do just that. Again, the same scientific principles that got you this far will carry you into the future, and help you enjoy your new body for the rest of your life.

So when you're ready to get started, turn to Chapter 10 for the first day of the program. The next 28 days will begin to transform your life and your health in very positive ways.

10

TAKING IT OFF:
THE CONDITIONING PHASE

Our 28-day Conditioning Phase contains specific assignments for you to do each day. To get the full weight-loss benefits, you must follow every step of the program. That's what it takes to recondition your body and override your weight regulator's upward pressure on your weight.

The conditioning process has five crucial steps:

1. Establishing conscious contact with your weight-regulating system

2. Reregulating the fat content in your diet

3. Reregulating your energy expenditure

4. Reregulating your eating behaviors

5. Conscious monitoring

Each of these steps is significant on its own, but together they act synergistically to create a far greater impact. In the pages that follow, we'll present the precise 28-day program you need to follow. For starters, at the beginning of each month, tear out one of the perforated color charts found in the book. Post the chart on the refrigerator or other place and, at the end of each day, fill it in according to these guidelines: Fill in the entire circle if you completely met your goal; fill in half the circle if you partially met the goal; leave the circle blank if you did not meet any of your goal. Now, before starting Day 1, remember these daily guidelines:

- *Read the daily section.*
- *Follow the day's assignments.*
- *Chart your progress.*

DAY 1

REDUCING FAT INTAKE

Fat: The Biggest Culprit in Your Diet

Your body is designed to preferentially burn carbohydrates for fuel before it begins burning fat. Thus, if you overeat dietary fat, you are much more likely to become fatter than if you overeat carbohydrates, because the excess fat you consume is more likely to be stored in your fat cells (or adipose tissue), where it will gradually add extra pounds to your body (see Day 19, page 202, for more details about this process).

Eating lots of fat can make weight loss an uphill fight for other reasons, too. Fats are a more concentrated source of calories than carbohydrates or protein. While each gram of fat supplies nine calories, a gram of carbohydrate or protein provides just four calories. If you prefer to work with pounds, one pound of pure dietary fat supplies 4,086 calories; one pound of pure carbohydrate or pure protein supplies 1,816 calories. Ounce for ounce, pound for pound, if you substitute carbohydrate for fat, you'll end up consuming fewer calories, even if you continue to eat the same amount of food (by weight) as you did before. In my own case, once I started concentrating on fat instead of calories, the volume of food I ate actually increased significantly while my weight went down.

What's the bottom line? Excess dietary fat makes you fat. You gain weight because you consume more fat than your body requires for energy. To lose those extra pounds and keep them off, you need to cut down on the fat in your diet.

Our system uses a simple law of averages to keep your total fat intake at 20 percent or less of your calorie consumption. Here's how it works:

- You will significantly increase your intake of foods that have 10 percent or less of their calories in the form of fat. While I won't go so far as to say you can eat unlimited quantities of these low-fat foods, I promise that you can eat enough of them to feel fully satisfied all of the time—probably enough to feel stuffed.

- You will cut back drastically on foods that get 30 percent or more of their calories from fat. Even though no foods are forbidden in our program, this group of foods does not belong on the list of choices you consume regularly.

- You will eat the remaining foods (which get from 11 to 29 percent of their calories from fat) thoughtfully and carefully.

Using this system, you should find yourself consuming a diet that is at or below a 20 percent fat level, thanks to the law of averages. When you are at that level, you will begin to lose weight, and you will be much more likely to keep it off.

In the material that follows, we'll explain in more detail how simply this system works, in lieu of the multiple-step calculations that are necessary when you're counting fat grams. This method is all you need to know to help put this weight-loss program into action.

THE LAW OF AVERAGES

There are several ways to reach your goal of a diet that gets only 20 percent of its calories from fat:

- You could eat only foods that contain exactly 20 percent fat (I'm only kidding; this would be an impossible task).

- You could determine precisely how many calories you consume each day, then determine how many grams of fat would equal 20 percent of that number, and then eat that precise amount of fat (this is possible, but it involves so much work and record-keeping, it is not practical for most busy people).

- You could use "the law of averages" to do the work for you (this is the method I use and recommend to others; read on to see how you can make it work for you).

We use the law of averages all the time in our daily lives. When driving a car, we use it to determine that our average speed on a trip will be about 45 miles an hour if half our time is spent on roads with a 35 miles-per-hour speed limit and the other half is spent on roads that allow us to drive at 55 miles an hour. When purchasing stocks, we know that our average price per share will be about $50 if we bought a third of the shares we own at that price, a third at about $40, and a third at about $60. Few of us would worry about being off in our calculations by a few miles per hour or a dollar or two in the cost of our shares. It's just not worth the time it would take to be more precise.

The same thing is true when calculating the fat content of your diet. If you eat as much as you can of foods that are very low in fat (10 percent fat calories or less), and you eat little or no food that is higher than 30 percent fat, the law of averages will keep your total fat intake at about the 20 percent level (usually, between 15 and 20 percent). Even if you eat a little butter once in a while (100 percent fat calories) or a couple of slices of bacon (about 80 percent fat calories) or even a scoop of ice cream (about 50 percent fat calories), the law of averages will be on your side if you also ate some nonfat foods that day. It's as simple as that.

Using this approach means you can lose weight without a rigid diet. It means there will not have to be any forbidden foods. Because, with this approach, you can balance out any high-fat food you eat with some good low-fat and nonfat choices.

Be aware, however, that the law of averages does not permit you to eat an unlimited amount of low-fat foods. If you do that, your daily caloric intake will quickly exceed the amount of calories you burn, and your excess fat calories will be added to the fat that is already stored in your body.

So, to repeat, I'd like you to use the following set of guidelines when selecting foods to eat. These guidelines will help ensure that, by the end of each day, only 20 percent—or less—of the calories you've consumed will come from fat.

- Significantly increase your intake of foods that derive 10 percent or less of their calories from fat.

- Cut back drastically on foods that get 30 percent or more of their calories from fat.

- Eat thoughtfully and carefully those foods which get 11 to 29 percent of their calories from fat.

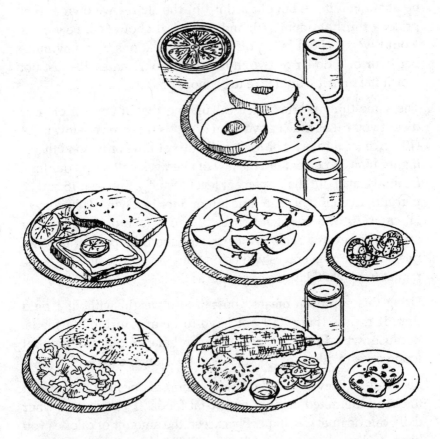

This illustration shows how the "law of averages" will keep your overall daily fat intake at the right level. It depicts the foods listed on page 89, eaten over the course of a day. Although these foods vary in fat content, when taken collectively, the law of averages has kept the total fat calories at less than 11 percent—a very desirable level when weight loss is your goal.

THE LAW OF AVERAGES: AN EXAMPLE

Here's an example of how the law of averages works, using foods consumed by an individual in a typical day:

"10 PERCENT OR LESS" FOODS

BAGEL (195 calories/5% from fat) *10 fat calories*

2 TSP. JAM (40 calories/0% from fat) *0 fat calories*

3 8-OUNCE GLASSES OF SKIM MILK (240 calories/4% from fat) *10 fat calories*

½ GRAPEFRUIT (50 calories/2% from fat) *1 fat calorie*

APPLE (80 calories/5% from fat) *4 fat calories*

2 LARGE PRETZELS (200 calories/0% from fat) *0 fat calories*

1 CUP OF BROWN RICE (220 calories/7% from fat) *16 fat calories*

CORN ON THE COB (one ear) (80 calories/10% from fat) *8 fat calories*

½ CUCUMBER (20 calories/10% from fat) *2 fat calories*

2 TBSP. FAT-FREE ITALIAN DRESSING (15 calories/0% from fat) *0 fat calories*

"11 TO 29 PERCENT" FOODS

2 SLICES SANDWICH BREAD (140 calories/12% from fat) *17 fat calories*

3 OZ. 97% FAT-FREE TURKEY LUNCHEON MEAT (90 calories/24% from fat) *22 fat calories*

8 OZ. CHICKEN BREAST (250 calories/12% from fat) *30 fat calories*

¼ HEAD LETTUCE (20 calories/15% from fat) *3 fat calories*

TOMATO (26 calories/12% from fat) *3 fat calories*

"30 PERCENT OR MORE" FOODS

2 CHOCOLATE CHIP COOKIES (160 calories/45% from fat) *72 fat calories*

Total caloric intake for the day   1,826

Total calories from fat for the day   198 (less than 11%)

DAY I

Assignment

1. Decrease fat in your diet so it accounts for less than 20 percent of your total calories for the day. To accomplish this, increase your intake of foods that have 10 percent or less of their calories from fat—and cut back significantly on foods with 30 percent or more of their calories from fat.

2. Cover 500 feet (walking or running at any pace, continuously or in smaller segments).

3. Walk up one flight of stairs.

4. Eat your meals using the pacing system, pausing 30 seconds between each bite.

5. Eat at least three meals.

6. Choose one of the following:

   a. Replace one high-fat product in your kitchen with a low- or nonfat product (examples: nonfat yogurt or sorbet in place of ice cream; nonfat cereal in place of one that contains fat).

   b. Categorize the foods in one of your cupboards into nonfat, low-fat and high-fat foods. Categorizing them will help you make good food choices quickly.

7. Put your Self-Monitoring tearout chart (from the back of the book) on your refrigerator door. Score yourself at the end of the day for goals accomplished.

DAY 2

EXERCISE & WEIGHT LOSS

If I had to pick a single issue that could predict your chance of long-term success with our program (or any other program), I would select "exercise." Although every element in our program is important, the research clearly shows that people who are physically active—especially those who engage in regular exercise—are much more likely to lose weight and keep it off than sedentary people. All of the weight loss experts with whom I have spoken agree: Stopping exercise is the first sign that people will gain back the weight they've lost.

Interestingly enough, it probably isn't just the effect that exercise has on the number of calories you are burning. It's the fact that once the exercise "goes," many people quickly give up the other essential elements of their program.

In Chapter 6, I discussed all of the reasons why your weight-loss (and fitness) program should include daily exercise. To ensure that you translate my message into action, this 28-day Conditioning Phase contains a very specific and mandatory exercise assignment every day. If you follow these assignments to the letter (or substitute other physical activities of equivalent value), I'm confident that you will see and feel how essential this part of the program is to your continued success. I believe you will also enjoy the exercise.

The exercise assignments in this book are the minimum amount you should do each day, so don't feel limited by them if you feel like doing more (and you are medically capable of doing more). And don't be afraid to change the assignments to other activities you like better. Let's be realistic: You're not going to stick with an exercise program over the long-term if you're not enjoying it. So look for ways to add fun at the same time you are adding activity.

In the material that follows (and in the days that follow), you'll find more information you can use to develop an exercise program that works well for you. If you need more help in this area, get it. You'll find expert help at your local "Y" or at a commercial fitness center that uses certified instructors. Talk to your doctor about the best kind of exercise for you. The more you learn about exercise, the more you'll enjoy it and benefit from it.

Aerobic Exercise

Any activity that forces you to breathe deeply and use your major muscles in a continuous and rhythmic fashion for more than 12 to 15 minutes can be used to improve aerobic fitness. Aerobic training increases the amount of physical work you can do, and speeds your recovery afterward. Aerobic training also increases the efficiency of your heart, so it does not have to beat as rapidly to get the same task done.

During an aerobic workout, your body burns calories faster as your muscles work harder. Aerobic exercise not only burns more calories during the activity, but also causes your metabolism to maintain a more rapid rate for some time afterward. Studies have shown that a person's metabolic rate can remain elevated for 20 minutes to an hour after exercise. What's more, after about 30 minutes of continual aerobic exercise at low to moderate intensity, the body increases its reliance on fat stores for energy (at higher intensities, it draws on carbohydrates).

You can choose from numerous aerobic activities, several of which are described below. Others worth mentioning include jumping rope, using a trampoline, roller blading, ice skating, and dancing. If cardiovascular aerobic fitness is your goal, you must work out at least 20 minutes, four times a week, at an intensity level high enough to raise your heart rate to 50 to 70 percent of its maximum. (Determine your maximum heart rate by subtracting your age from 220. If you are 40 years old, your maximum heart rate is 180; so you should exercise in the range of 90 to 126 beats per minute to remain in your target zone of 50 to 70 percent of maximum.)

When weight loss is your goal, however, it is not necessary to exercise at such high levels. You'd be better off with longer sessions of lower intensity every day.

Whatever activity or mix of activities you choose, exercise can make a remarkable improvement in the way you look and feel. Once you become—as I predict you will—"hooked" on exercise, you may find yourself seeking out new activities to try. (See the chart titled "Approximate Calories Burned During Various Activities" on page 95. It will help you determine the amount of calories you can burn with various aerobic activities.)

WALKING

Walking is an ideal activity for weight loss. Walking is easy to do, isn't limited by your age or geographic location, can be done without expensive facilities or equipment, and doesn't require professional instruction or supervision. Walking can also improve your aerobic fitness level if you maintain a pace brisk enough to get your heart rate in the target zone—50 to 70 percent of maximum.

Regular walking enhances your endurance by increasing the capacity of your lungs to move air in and out and by improving the strength and efficiency of the muscles in your legs, abdomen, and back. An additional benefit of walking is that people who are overweight or out of shape can walk farther than they can run; being able to go the extra distance makes it possible to burn more calories. For both weight management and aerobic fitness, walking fits the bill perfectly.

Walking can be done at a number of levels, ranging from an easy stroll (about one to two miles per hour) to striding or race walking (about five miles per hour). A good pace to shoot for is three to four miles per hour. At this pace, walking burns about 300 to 400 calories per hour.

In our program, you'll be required to cover a specified distance each day. The first day, you walked 500 feet (about the length of a city block), and each day after that you will add another 500 feet. For example, your assignment today is to walk 1,000 feet. By the end of the 28-day program, you will be walking 14,000 feet (or about three miles) a day.

Keep in mind, however, that you don't have to walk the entire assigned distance all at once. You can divide it into two, five, ten, or as many segments as you like during the day, and you will achieve the same benefits.

RUNNING

Obviously, running places more demands on your body than walking, making the aerobic workout more intense. If your beginning fitness level is low—because you've been inactive for years—you'll be better off starting with a walking program. But for people who are already at an appropriate fitness level, running is an excellent choice. Compared to walking, running provides the same cardiovascular conditioning and weight control benefits in about half the time. (Running at about six miles per hour burns roughly 600 calories per hour.)

A significant drawback of running is the increased risk of injury, especially to the knees and other joints. Joggers need to take particular care in selecting shoes that provide support while absorbing shock.

SWIMMING AND OTHER WATER EXERCISES

Swimming is one of the best exercises for overall body conditioning. It is also one of the safer aerobic exercise choices. Swimming is an impact-free activity; it does not stress bones and joints. Also, unlike running, walking, and cycling, swimming builds upper body strength. What's more, many people associate water and swimming pools with fun, so they are more likely to stick with a swimming program. Swimming at a steady crawl burns more than 500 calories per hour.

Besides swimming, other aerobic exercises that can be done in water include water walking and water aerobics. Water walking—which involves walking from one side of a pool's shallow end to the other against the resistance that the water provides—is an excellent way to condition leg muscles. In water aerobics, people do repetitive leg

APPROXIMATE CALORIES BURNED
DURING VARIOUS ACTIVITIES

(calories burned per minute)

Activity	Weight			
	130 lb	150 lb	170 lb	200 lb
Basketball	8.0	9.5	11.0	12.5
Carpentry	3.0	3.5	4.0	5.0
Car wash and wax	3.5	4.0	4.5	5.0
Cleaning	4.0	4.5	5.0	6.0
Football	8.0	9.0	10.0	12.0
Gardening	3.0–8.0	4.0–9.0	4.0–10.0	5.0–12.0
Golf	5.0	6.0	7.0	8.0
Hiking	7.0	8.5	9.5	10.5
Horseback riding (trot)	6.5	7.5	8.5	10.0
Jumping rope (80 jumps/min)	10.0	11.0	12.5	14.5
Mowing lawn (hand mower)	6.5	7.5	8.5	9.5
Racquetball	10.5	12.0	13.5	16.5
Shoveling snow	7.0	8.0	9.0	11.0
Skating	7.0	8.0	9.0	11.0
Skiing	7.0	8.0	9.0	11.0
Squash	12.5	14.0	16.0	19.5
Stair climbing	6.0	7.0	8.0	10.0
Tennis	6.5	7.5	8.5	10.0
Walking (3 mph)	3.5	4.0	4.5	5.0
(4 mph)	5.0	6.0	6.5	7.5

and arm movements while standing in the water. Check with your local YMCA or public pool to see if it offers these classes.

CYCLING

Riding a bicycle is another effective aerobic exercise. It raises your heart rate and develops lower body strength. Cycling also offers the pleasures of changing scenery, fresh air, and a sense of speed. But the risk of injury is much higher than with some other aerobic activities, especially if you ride through busy city streets. In some locations (like city streets) bicyclists must stop frequently, so the aerobic benefits are impeded. If you choose bicycling as your aerobic activity, be sure to wear a good helmet and plan a route through safe, less traveled roads. Bicycling at ten miles per hour burns about 400 calories per hour.

AEROBICS CLASSES

Most health clubs offer a variety of aerobics classes, including aerobic dance, low-impact aerobics, and step aerobics. All involve performing repetitive movements—such as arm swings, leg lifts, and dance steps—to the beat of rhythmic music. Low-impact classes reduce the risk of leg strain and injury because in all the moves, at least one foot remains on the floor. Step aerobics, which is mostly low-impact movement, uses low benches, roughly 4 to 12 inches high, to accentuate the aerobic and muscle-building effect of the movements. Depending on the intensity, an hour of aerobics will burn off between 400 and 600 calories.

Many people are stimulated by the energetic atmosphere and group support of aerobics classes. You may even find the sheer fun of dancing to music so exhilarating that the exercise becomes not only physically beneficial but also emotionally uplifting and satisfying. If you decide to start taking aerobics classes, make sure you find a reputable health club or dance studio staffed by certified instructors.

STATIONARY EXERCISE MACHINES

Stationary machines—bicycles, rowing machines, stair climbers, treadmills, cross-country ski simulators—are another fine choice for aerobic exercise. They provide most of the same benefits as the original activity they are modeled after, but offer an added advantage: You don't have to contend with real-world obstacles, such as foul weather, traffic, and stoplights. Also, if you have a machine at home, you can work out while watching the TODAY show or the evening news.

EXERCISE VIDEOTAPES

Since the video exercise boom started in the 1980s, literally hundreds of home exercise programs have been produced. It seems as though every major—and minor—star in Hollywood has come out with a tape in the last few years. Most of these programs are designed and overseen by professionals in the exercise field, so the risk of injury is minimal. Most video stores rent exercise tapes, so you can try them before committing to a purchase. It's a good idea to purchase several different exercise videos so you can vary your routines. Be sure to purchase programs that are appropriate to your current fitness level. Don't worry about outgrowing them as your fitness level improves. You can always use your easier programs on days when you want a lighter workout.

Strength Training

Aerobic conditioning is only one part of the exercise program we've designed for you. The other is strength training. Aerobic exercises work your muscles repetitively, causing your heart to pump faster and your oxygen intake to increase. Strength training works your muscles against resistance to increase their tone and strength.

Because working with weights does not put the muscles through nearly as much motion and repetition as aerobic exercise, strength training burns fewer calories (roughly 300 per hour). Even so, there's an important reason to include strength training in your weight-loss program: Strength training helps you preserve your muscles. Remember, muscles burn calories faster than fat, so it is essential to protect them when you are losing weight.

A series of strength-training exercises is described below. These exercises will work most of the major muscle groups of your upper body, including your biceps (front of your upper arm), triceps (back of your upper arm), deltoids (shoulders), and pectoralis muscles (chest). Exercises targeting the muscles of your lower body are not included as they should be strengthened sufficiently by your walking and stair climbing assignments.

Contrary to what many people believe, initiating a weight-training program does not require a huge investment. For these exercises, you can work out with one-pound food cans, cloth sacks filled with sand, quart- or gallon-size plastic bottles filled with water or sand, or inexpensive barbells, which can be purchased from any athletic store.

To get you started, we've created a very unique equipment system that uses an ordinary bucket as a carrier for cans or sacks of food (do not use glass containers and don't fill the bucket with water or other liquids). As your strength improves, you can gradually increase the weight of the bucket by adding half-pound or one-pound cans or sacks. Do not fill the bucket with weights that exceed the strength of the bucket or its handle.

We've illustrated several specific strength-training exercises you can do to protect your muscles. Though the equipment may appear makeshift and amateurish, your muscles can't distinguish the weight in the buckets from the most expensive set of weights sold in the store. As you get stronger, you should give serious consideration to purchasing a more professional set of weights or joining a fitness facility that has weight-lifting equipment.

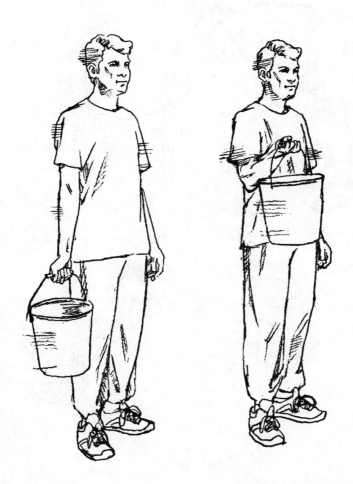

ARM CURL
Muscles strengthened:
Biceps

Exercise:
Grasp the bucket in your hand, palm facing forward, elbow at your side, and arm straight. While standing up straight, slowly lift the bucket by bending the elbow, and pause momentarily when the edge of the bucket touches your forearm. Then slowly lower the bucket to the starting position.

Tip:
When lifting, keep your elbow firmly in place against your side. Do not swing your body to help raise the bucket.

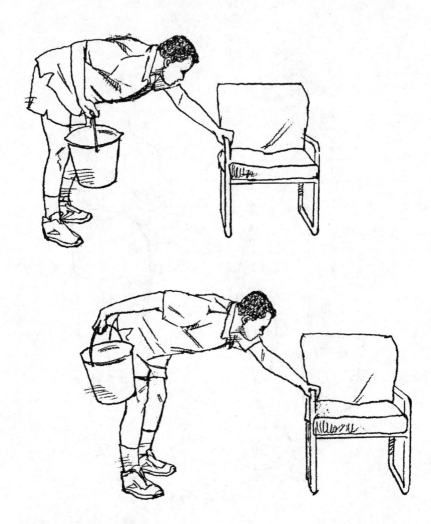

TRICEPS EXTENSION
Muscles strengthened:
Triceps

Exercise:
While keeping your legs and back nearly straight, bend forward at the hips, raise your head and look forward. As one hand rests on a chair or table, grasp the bucket handle with the other hand, keeping your palm facing the direction in which you are looking. Keep your elbow firmly at your side, and allow the bucket to hang comfortably toward the floor. Next, slowly straighten the arm behind you, lifting the weight as you do. Then return to the starting position.

Tip:
By resting one arm on a table or chair, you will take strain off your lower back.

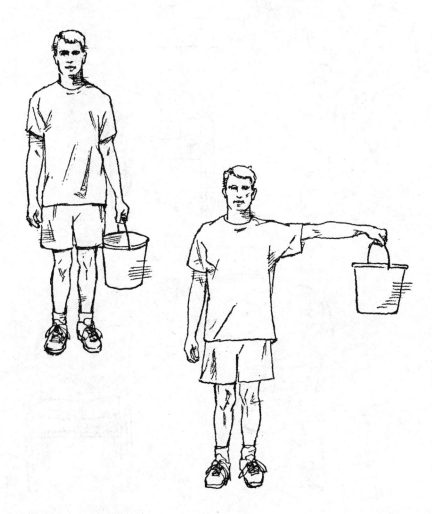

STRAIGHT ARM RAISE
Muscles strengthened:
Shoulder muscles

Exercise:
With your palms facing your body, grasp the pail handle, and allow the pail to hang comfortably at your side. Stand up straight with your shoulders back, and slowly lift your arm to the side (keeping your elbow straight) until your arm is parallel to the floor or just a little higher. Then lower the weight slowly to the starting position.

Tip:
To resist the temptation to swing the weight up and down rapidly, force yourself to pause for just a moment with the weight in the highest position.

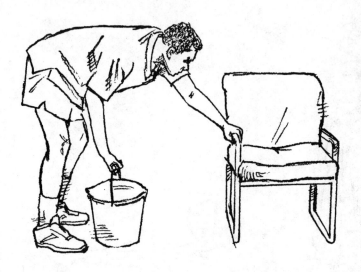

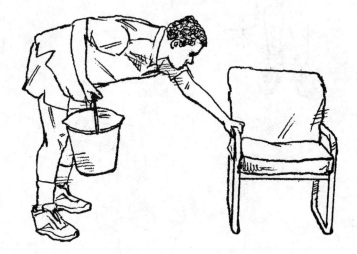

BENT-OVER ROW
Muscles strengthened:
Back muscles, biceps

Exercise:
With your legs and back kept nearly straight, bend forward at the hips, raise your head and look forward. As one hand rests on a chair or table, grasp the bucket handle in your other hand, palm facing your body, and allow the bucket to hang free. Lift the bucket slowly until the handle touches your side, pause briefly, and lower slowly to the starting position.

Tip:
By keeping one arm on a table or chair, you'll take strain off your lower back.

ADVANCED

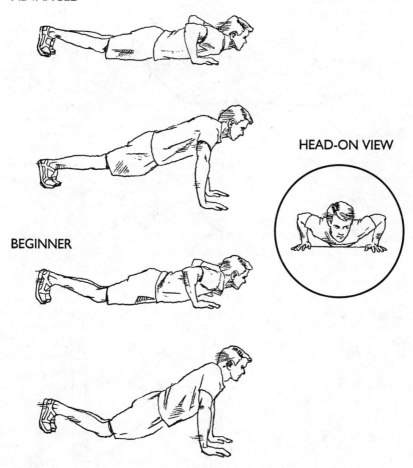

HEAD-ON VIEW

BEGINNER

PUSH-UPS
Muscles strengthened:
The muscles connecting the chest wall to the bones of the upper arm and shoulder; triceps.

Exercise:
Lie on the floor on your stomach, with your hands flat on the floor just to the sides of your shoulders. Straighten your arms until your chest is one inch off the floor. Raise your head, look forward, and keep your back straight as you push up until your elbows are straight. Then lower yourself by bending the elbows, stopping when your chest is one inch off the floor.

Tip:
When you first begin doing push-ups, keep your knees on the floor at all times; as you become stronger, let only your toes and hands touch the floor, while keeping your entire body straight.

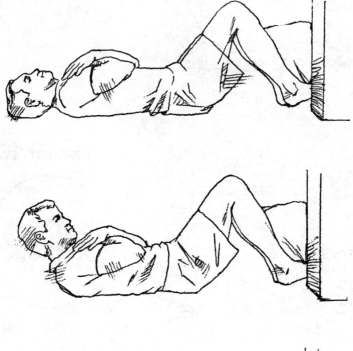

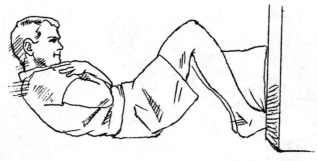

SIT-UPS
Muscles strengthened:
Abdominal muscles

Exercise:
Lie on your back with your knees bent comfortably (place your feet under a bed or chair if you like). With your arms folded loosely across your chest, raise your upper body until your shoulder blades are off the floor. Pause for a moment, then lower your body to the floor.

Tip:
Have a friend hold your feet in place to keep them from rising during each sit-up.

Stair Climbing

We've made stair climbing, along with walking, an important element of our program, not just to burn calories, but also to strengthen leg muscles, which helps preserve lean body tissues as you lose weight. You'll be asked to climb one flight of stairs a day for the first week; two a day for the second; three per day for the third week; and four flights each day thereafter. Climbing stairs will also quickly raise your heart rate and—if you're strong enough to keep climbing for a while—improve your aerobic conditioning.

However, even if you're in pretty good shape, you may have trouble making it up more than three or four flights of stairs at one time. What is it about stairs that makes them so difficult to climb? You're working directly against the force of gravity, and that uses up a lot of energy (which explains why stair climbing burns so many calories).

The trouble is, most of us have become experts at avoiding stairs. We've gotten so spoiled with elevators and escalators that even one flight of stairs seems like too much to handle. And that's another reason why we've included stair climbing in your daily assignments—to recondition the way you think about stairs. In fact, to keep up with the assignments, you may have to go out of your way to find stairs to climb.

If you live in a home with no stairs, here are some ideas to help you complete your daily climbing assignments:

- Walk each day to your local high school stadium and walk up and down the bleachers repetitively, just like the athletes do.

- Visit your local shopping mall or a nearby office building and use the stairwells instead of the elevators.

Don't look for excuses; look for stairs.

DAY 2

Assignment

1. Decrease fat in your diet so that it accounts for less than 20 percent of your total calories for the day. To accomplish this, increase your intake of foods that have 10 percent or less of their calories from fat and cut back significantly on foods with 30 percent or more of their calories from fat.

2. Cover 1,000 feet (walking or running at any pace, continuously or in smaller segments).

3. Walk up one flight of stairs.

4. Eat your meals using the pacing system, pausing 30 seconds between each bite.

5. Eat at least three meals.

6. Choose one of the following:

   a. Engage in a physical activity that you usually pass up. For example, use the stairs in the office instead of the elevator or play an outdoor game.

   b. Form a walking club with friends. Make plans to walk together at least once a week (preferably more often).

7. Using your Self-Monitoring tearout chart, score yourself at the end of the day for goals accomplished.

DAY 3

BEHAVIOR MODIFICATION: PACING

The way to begin changing your eating behavior is by increasing your awareness of the way you eat now. In my opinion, the most important behavior to start with is your eating speed. Most rapid eaters have no idea how quickly they race through their meals. Ask them how much time elapses between their bites of food, and they'll guess somewhere between 15 and 30 seconds. But if you actually watch them eat and time the intervals between their bites (don't tell them you're doing it), you'll find that they are putting a new bite into their mouth every five to ten seconds. At that rate, they'll consume a huge amount of food before their brain can recognize that satiation has occurred, and send a signal to stop eating.

No matter how much food you consume, it takes your brain about 20 minutes to recognize that you have eaten enough to satisfy your body's needs. People who eat slowly will consume less food during this 20-minute period and feel just as satisfied as will faster eaters who consume much more in the same time frame. Unfortunately, this mechanism for recognizing satiety may not work in some obese people, so they never get the feeling of being full. Therefore, they may continue to eat for a much longer period of time. Even so, if they slow their eating pace, they will consume much less food during whatever period of time they are eating.

Slowing the pace at which you eat can not only reduce your food intake, but also increase your enjoyment of food. By taking the time to savor the taste of your food and appreciate its aroma, texture, and appearance, you make the process of eating more satisfying. If you learn to derive more pleasure from eating this way, you should be able to end each meal feeling more satisfied with less food.

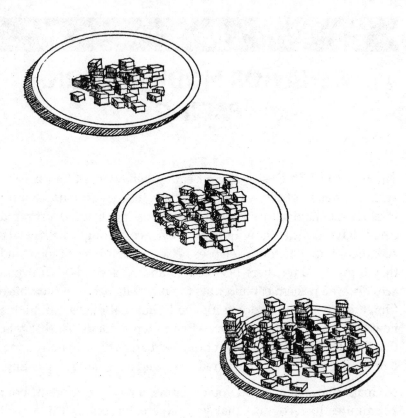

These three plates show the amount of food you'd consume in 20 minutes at varying eating speeds, and the importance of slowing your pace. The first plate has 40 cubes (each represents a bite of food), indicating how much food you'd eat in 20 minutes when pausing 30 seconds between bites. The second plate, with 80 cubes, shows the number of bites in the same time period when a new bite is taken every 15 seconds. The third plate has 160 cubes, which is the number of bites you'd take in 20 minutes when pausing only 7.5 seconds between bites.

The Pacing Program

In the following pages, you will learn a pacing technique that can help you learn much more about the way you now eat. If you eat too rapidly, it will help you slow the pace. With regular practice, this pacing technique will help you replace your current eating patterns with new ones that will make it easier for you to overcome the upward pressure of your weight regulator.

Although this pacing technique doesn't work for everyone, it has helped me personally, and we have received glowing reports from others who have used it. We offered an audiocassette version of my pacing program on television, and within weeks of our first sales, calls were pouring in to the network from people who wanted to share their good results.

One of the most exciting reports came from Sue and Ted Clark, a Sacramento, California couple who used the pacing program and lost a total of 167 pounds together. Sue said that when she first tried the program, she was astonished to discover how fast she and Ted had been eating. Using the pacing techniques and affirmations in the audiotape, Sue and Ted learned to eat more slowly and really enjoy their food. After years of countless diets, something about this program "clicked" for Sue, and enabled her to lose 107 pounds (Ted lost 60). She enthusiastically credits all of their success to pacing, but I think that their new walking routine (also part of the program you are starting now) deserves some of the credit, too.

I can't promise that the pacing program will make everyone lose as much weight as Ted and Sue, but of one thing I am fairly certain: If you use this program just once, you will become more aware of your eating behaviors than ever before, and if you are a rapid eater you'll be shocked into working on your eating speed. Use this pacing program for 28 days, and eating more slowly will become an almost automatic part of your behavior. Your mind and body will become so conditioned by the pacing program that you'll slow your eating pace without even thinking about it. Not only that, you'll enjoy your meals more than ever before.

There are four key elements in the pacing program: a relaxation exercise, a hunger test, a pacing system for eating, and a set of affirmations that help you to make cognitive changes.

THE RELAXATION EXERCISE

The relaxation exercise sets the tone for the meal and eliminates stressful sensations that make you eat even when you're not hungry. This part of the program contains a short and simple deep breathing technique you can use before you eat, anytime and anywhere. In less than a minute, it will calm your mind and body and cancel some of the tension and stress you may be feeling. If you are about to eat as a reaction to tension and stress, the relaxation technique may help you overcome the urge to eat. Most people respond automatically to relaxation by eating more slowly.

THE HUNGER TEST

This portion of the program is designed to help you differentiate whether you are eating because you are truly hungry, or whether other factors—such as situational or psychological issues—are creating urges that make you want to eat. Although it is very difficult for some people to distinguish between so-called biologic hunger and emotional hunger, consciously examining the situation can make the process easier. This portion of the program contains some simple questions that will help you determine what is triggering your desire to eat at any particular time.

What does true, biologic hunger feel like? Hunger pangs—those gnawing sensations felt in or around the stomach—are a good indication of true hunger. Hunger pangs are a signal that it's okay to start eating. But some people don't feel true hunger pangs until several hours after their last meal—or not at all. If hunger pangs are not present, you can still eat—but only if you have really thought about it, and have consciously decided it's the right thing to do.

Once you have started eating, it is just as important to stop when the physical signs of hunger are gone. (Do not confuse this with the feeling of being "stuffed," which means that you have eaten too much.)

THE PACING SYSTEM

This portion of the program is designed to slow down your eating, and to help you feel more satisfied with less food. Eating more slowly helps you in several ways. You will have consumed less food by the time your brain recognizes that you are no longer hungry. You will have more time to enjoy the various sensory pleasures that good food has to offer (taste, smell, consistency). You will also have time to think about what you are eating and why. If you are eating too quickly, you miss the best part of eating. The taste, smell, sight, and texture of your food can provide you with additional sensations that will make you feel just as satisfied—if not more satisfied—with less food. If you use the pacing system regularly, enjoyment of these other pleasures will soon come automatically.

The pacing system is contained in a script that can be read out loud or silently to yourself while you eat. The time it takes to read the script will automatically space out your bites of food to intervals of approximately 25 to 30 seconds. You can take as many bites of food as you wish, and you can eat for as long as you want, as long as you maintain this interval between bites.

IS SKIPPING MEALS HAZARDOUS TO YOUR HEALTH?

Some people believe that one of the best strategies for losing weight is skipping meals. They don't eat breakfast, or they work through their lunch hour, figuring that they're avoiding large numbers of calories that way.

Two things can go wrong if you use this strategy. First, hunger can lead to rebound eating—excessive food intake later in the day—which can sabotage your weight-loss plan. Second, if you skip meals, your resting metabolic rate will tend to decrease. If that happens, you'll burn fewer calories throughout the day, and you'll lose everything you "gained" by skipping the meals.

Of course, everyone is different. Some people never eat breakfast, whether or not they're dieting; they're just not hungry in the morning, and they eat normally the rest of the day without problems. Others, however, may skip breakfast, but by 10:30 become so hungry that they grab a midmorning snack of two doughnuts, or they overeat at lunch.

My advice is simple: If you skip meals and then find yourself gorging later, put yourself on a schedule of three to four meals a day (or three meals plus a snack). If your stomach is growling for food and you still deny yourself, you may pay the price by rebound eating. If you're skipping meals and seem to fare just fine, though, it's probably all right to continue doing so. But I still suggest that you try eating three meals a day, and see how that pattern works for you.

THE AFFIRMATIONS

This portion of the program is designed to counter the negative beliefs and attitudes that many overweight people harbor about themselves and about their ability to manage their weight problem effectively. The program contains a series of affirmations that increase awareness of these issues and counteract negative thoughts by substituting more positive and constructive statements. These affirmations condition your mind and body to react in a more healthful way to food, while helping keep your weight in proper perspective. The affirmations will also help you get more enjoyment out of food and eating.

HOW FAST DO YOU EAT?

Before using this program, you should first take a moment to become more aware of the rate at which you usually eat. Set a timer for two minutes and count the number of bites you take during that time. Do the best you can to eat at your usual pace (this can be very difficult when you know you are timing yourself). Time an entire meal to see how long it takes you from start to finish. You may be surprised to find your plate clean in only eight to ten minutes.

Another way to evaluate your eating speed is to compare yourself to others. When eating with family and friends, pay attention to how quickly you finish your meal relative to the others. When you are eating out, discreetly compare your eating pace to that of other diners. You'll probably notice a great variation in the pace at which other people eat. Try to identify the fastest and slowest eaters in your line of sight. Where do you fit in? Next time you're on an airplane, take a look around when food is being served. Some passengers will have their trays cleared in less than five minutes, but the slow eaters will still be eating long after most of the trays are gone. What will you be doing?

If you have children in the house, observe how you eat as a family. Is one person setting a fast pace that everyone is trying to follow? Are you repeating patterns that you learned in childhood? Are your children repeating your eating patterns?

The Script

You can use the pacing program in two ways: (a) read the script that follows as you eat your meals, or (b) record an audiotape from the script that follows, and listen to it as you eat. Here is the script to use:

Close your eyes and take a few deep breaths—slowly and gently. Breathe in through your nose and slowly fill your lungs as full as you can with air. As you breathe in, say to yourself, silently, "I am," and as you breathe out, say to yourself, silently, "relaxed." With each breath in and out, say to yourself, "I am . . . relaxed." And with each breath, allow yourself to become just a little more relaxed. Do this three or four times.

"I am relaxed."

"I am relaxed."

"I am relaxed."

Slowly open your eyes, and get ready to enjoy your meal.

From now on, you will eat only when you are hungry. Say to yourself, silently or out loud:

"From now on, I will eat only when I am hungry."

Say it three more times:

"From now on, I will eat only when I am hungry."

"From now on, I will eat only when I am hungry."

"From now on, I will eat only when I am hungry."

Before you eat anything, pause to be sure that you are really hungry— sure that the reason you are eating is to satisfy hunger.

Ask yourself, "Am I really hungry? Or is it something else I am feeling?" If you are not hungry—leave the table now. If you are hungry, take your first bite, but chew it slowly.

From now on, you will enjoy every aspect of the eating experience. You will enjoy the sight of your food, the taste of it, the texture, the aroma. You will enjoy everything about eating.

If you're chewing too quickly, you'll miss the best part of eating. From now on, you are going to chew your food slowly. From now on, you will savor your food.

Say to yourself, silently or out loud:

> **"From now on, I will chew my food more slowly. I will savor my food."**

Say it three more times:

> **"From now on, I will chew my food more slowly. I will savor my food."**

> **"From now on, I will chew my food more slowly. I will savor my food."**

> **"From now on, I will chew my food more slowly. I will savor my food."**

Are you still hungry? If so, take another bite, and chew it slowly. If not, wait to take a bite until after you have gone through the next section.

From now on, you will eat slowly, so you can feel more satisfied with less food. You will concentrate more on the look and smell and taste of your food, and you'll enjoy things you never even noticed before.

Say to yourself, silently or out loud:

> **"From now on, I will eat slowly, and I will feel more satisfied with less food."**

Say it three more times:

> **"From now on, I will eat slowly, and I will feel more satisfied with less food."**

> **"From now on, I will eat slowly, and I will feel more satisfied with less food."**

> **"From now on, I will eat slowly, and I will feel more satisfied with less food."**

Are you still hungry? If so, take another bite, and chew it slowly. If not, wait to take a bite until after you have gone through the next section.

From now on, you are going to take pleasure from the way your food looks. Remember, the more you satisfy all of your senses, the less food it takes to satisfy your hunger. Pay attention to the way your food looks. Really concentrate on its appearance. From now on, you are going to take pleasure from the appearance of your food.

Say to yourself, silently or out loud:

> **"From now on, I am going to take pleasure from the appearance of my food."**

Say it three more times:

"From now on, I am going to take pleasure from the appearance of my food."

"From now on, I am going to take pleasure from the appearance of my food."

"From now on, I am going to take pleasure from the appearance of my food."

Are you still hungry? If so, take another bite, and chew it slowly. If not, wait to take a bite until after you have gone through the next section.

The more you satisfy all of your senses, the less food it takes to satisfy your hunger. From now on, you will delight in the fragrance of your food.

Say to yourself, silently or out loud:

"From now on, I will delight in the fragrance of my food."

Say it three more times:

"From now on, I will delight in the fragrance of my food."

"From now on, I will delight in the fragrance of my food."

"From now on, I will delight in the fragrance of my food."

Are you still hungry? If so, take another bite, and chew it slowly. If not, wait to take a bite until after you have gone through the next section.

The more you concentrate on the actual taste of your food, the more you will enjoy it. From now on, you will enjoy the taste of your food.

Say to yourself, silently or out loud:

"From now on, I will enjoy the taste of my food."

Say it three more times:

"From now on, I will enjoy the taste of my food."

"From now on, I will enjoy the taste of my food."

"From now on, I will enjoy the taste of my food."

Are you still hungry? If so, take another bite, and chew it slowly. If not, wait to take a bite until after you have gone through the next section.

The more you notice the taste, fragrance, and appearance of your food, the more you will enjoy the experience of eating. From now on, you will enjoy everything about eating.

Say to yourself, silently or out loud:

> **"From now on, I will enjoy everything about eating."**

Say it three more times:

> **"From now on, I will enjoy everything about eating."**

> **"From now on, I will enjoy everything about eating."**

> **"From now on, I will enjoy everything about eating."**

Are you still hungry? If so, take another bite, and chew it slowly. If not, wait to take a bite until after you have gone through the next section.

Concentrate even more on what you are eating. Focus in on the finest details. You'll enjoy things you never even noticed before about your food. And the more you enjoy your food, the more satisfied you will be with what you eat.

Say to yourself, silently or out loud:

> **"The more I enjoy my food, the more satisfied I will be with what I eat."**

Say it three more times:

> **"The more I enjoy my food, the more satisfied I will be with what I eat."**

> **"The more I enjoy my food, the more satisfied I will be with what I eat."**

> **"The more I enjoy my food, the more satisfied I will be with what I eat."**

Are you still hungry? If so, take another bite, and chew it slowly. If not, wait to take a bite until after you have gone through the next section.

The more satisfied you are with what you eat, the less you will eat.

Say to yourself, silently or out loud:

> **"The more satisfied I am with what I eat, the less I will eat."**

Say it three more times:

"The more satisfied I am with what I eat, the less I will eat."

"The more satisfied I am with what I eat, the less I will eat."

"The more satisfied I am with what I eat, the less I will eat."

Are you still hungry? If so, take another bite, and chew it slowly. If not, wait to take a bite until after you have gone through the next section.

You can eat anything you want now, because you are learning to control how much you eat. From now on, you can eat anything you want, because you will eat only when you are hungry.

Say to yourself, silently or out loud:

"From now on, I can eat anything I want, because I will eat only when I am hungry."

Say it three more times:

"From now on, I can eat anything I want, because I will eat only when I am hungry."

"From now on, I can eat anything I want, because I will eat only when I am hungry."

"From now on, I can eat anything I want, because I will eat only when I am hungry."

Are you still hungry? If so, take another bite, and chew it slowly. If not, wait to take a bite until after you have gone through the next section.

From now on, you will never feel deprived again because you can have anything you want to eat.

Say to yourself, silently or out loud:

"From now on, I will never feel deprived again, because I can have anything I want to eat."

Say it three more times:

"From now on, I will never feel deprived again, because I can have anything I want to eat."

"From now on, I will never feel deprived again, because I can have anything I want to eat."

"From now on, I will never feel deprived again, because I can have anything I want to eat."

Are you still hungry? If so, take another bite, and chew it slowly. If not, wait to take a bite until after you have gone through the next section.

From now on, you will not worry about your weight, because you will eat only when you are hungry.

Say to yourself, silently or out loud:

> **"I will not worry about my weight, because I will eat only when I am hungry."**

Say it three more times:

> **"I will not worry about my weight, because I will eat only when I am hungry."**

> **"I will not worry about my weight, because I will eat only when I am hungry."**

> **"I will not worry about my weight, because I will eat only when I am hungry."**

Are you still hungry? If so, take another bite, and chew it slowly. If not, wait to take a bite until after you have gone through the next section.

If you continue to eat this way, you will gradually get rid of the weight you want to lose. When you lose weight gradually, it stays off. From now on, you will be content to lose weight gradually. You will lose weight one ounce at a time.

Say to yourself, silently or out loud:

> **"From now on, I will be content to lose weight gradually. I will lose weight one ounce at a time."**

Say it three more times:

> **"From now on, I will be content to lose weight gradually. I will lose weight one ounce at a time."**

> **"From now on, I will be content to lose weight gradually. I will lose weight one ounce at a time."**

> **"From now on, I will be content to lose weight gradually. I will lose weight one ounce at a time."**

Are you still hungry? If so, take another bite, and chew it slowly. If not, wait to take a bite until after you have gone through the next section.

Ultimately, you will lose as much weight as you want to lose if you are patient. You will be patient, and you will lose weight.

Say to yourself, silently or out loud:

> **"I will be patient, and I will lose weight."**

Say it three more times:

> **"I will be patient, and I will lose weight."**

> **"I will be patient, and I will lose weight."**

> **"I will be patient, and I will lose weight."**

Are you still hungry? If so, take another bite, and chew it slowly. If not, wait to take a bite until after you have gone through the next section.

You may be tempted to keep eating just because there's still some food left on your plate. From now on, you will not eat food just because it's on your plate.

Say to yourself, silently or out loud:

> **"I will not eat food just because it is on my plate."**

Say it three more times:

> **"I will not eat food just because it is on my plate."**

> **"I will not eat food just because it is on my plate."**

> **"I will not eat food just because it is on my plate."**

Are you still hungry? If so, take another bite, and chew it slowly. If not, wait to take a bite until after you have gone through the next section.

It's nice to know that you can stop eating if you are no longer hungry, and that you can go on eating if you are still hungry. It's also nice to know that you can treat your body the way it should be treated, and still lose weight.

Say to yourself, silently or out loud:

> **"From now on, I will never do anything unhealthy to my body in order to lose weight."**

Say it three more times:

> **"From now on, I will never do anything unhealthy to my body in order to lose weight."**

> **"From now on, I will never do anything unhealthy to my body in order to lose weight."**

> **"From now on, I will never do anything unhealthy to my body in order to lose weight."**

Are you still hungry? If so, take another bite, and chew it slowly. If not, wait to take a bite until after you have gone through the next section.

When your weight becomes the overriding issue in your life, you begin to feel guilty or angry every time you eat. From now on, you will not feel guilty or angry about eating again.

Say to yourself, silently or out loud:

> **"From now on, I will not feel guilty or angry about eating again."**

Say it three more times:

> **"From now on, I will not feel guilty or angry about eating again."**

> **"From now on, I will not feel guilty or angry about eating again."**

> **"From now on, I will not feel guilty or angry about eating again."**

Are you still hungry? If so, take another bite, and chew it slowly. If not, wait to take a bite until after you have gone through the next section.

One of the problems we all face is the value our society places on a thin body. That's what pressures many of us to do the harmful things we do, in order to lose weight. From now on, you will stop placing so much emphasis on your weight.

Say to yourself, silently or out loud:

> **"From now on, I will stop placing so much emphasis on my weight."**

Say it three more times:

> **"From now on, I will stop placing so much emphasis on my weight."**

> **"From now on, I will stop placing so much emphasis on my weight."**

> **"From now on, I will stop placing so much emphasis on my weight."**

Are you still hungry? If so, take another bite, and chew it slowly. If not, wait to take a bite until after you have gone through the next section.

Most overweight people worry too much about what other people think about them. When you let other people use your weight to determine your worth, you never know who you are. Remember, you are not what people see on the surface. From now on, you will not lose weight to please other people.

Say to yourself, silently or out loud:

> **"I am not what people see on the surface, and I will not lose weight to please other people."**

Say it three more times:

> **"I am not what people see on the surface, and I will not lose weight to please other people."**

> **"I am not what people see on the surface, and I will not lose weight to please other people."**

> **"I am not what people see on the surface, and I will not lose weight to please other people."**

Are you still hungry? If so, take another bite, and chew it slowly. If not, wait to take a bite until after you have gone through the next section.

Some people place so much emphasis on their weight that they actually begin to confuse their weight on the scale with their self-worth. You are not your weight on the scale, and you will not measure your worth that way.

Say to yourself, silently or out loud:

> **"I am not my weight on the scale, and I will not measure my worth that way."**

Say it three more times:

> **"I am not my weight on the scale, and I will not measure my worth that way."**

> **"I am not my weight on the scale, and I will not measure my worth that way."**

> **"I am not my weight on the scale, and I will not measure my worth that way."**

Are you still hungry? If so, take another bite, and chew it slowly. If not, wait to take a bite until after you have gone through the next section.

When you let your self-worth fluctuate with your weight on the scale, you never know who you are. One day your weight is down, and you feel terrific. The next day, your weight is up, and you feel like a nothing. And all the while, you really have not changed at all. Remember, you are not your weight. You are a decent, attractive human being.

Say to yourself, silently or out loud:

"I am not my weight. I am a decent, attractive human being."

Say it three more times:

"I am not my weight. I am a decent, attractive human being."

"I am not my weight. I am a decent, attractive human being."

"I am not my weight. I am a decent, attractive human being."

Are you still hungry? If so, take another bite, and chew it slowly. If not, wait to take a bite until after you have gone through the next section.

From now on, you will listen to your body, and you will eat only when you are hungry.

Say to yourself, silently or out loud:

"From now on, I will listen to my body, and I will eat only when I am hungry."

Say it three more times:

"From now on, I will listen to my body, and I will eat only when I am hungry."

"From now on, I will listen to my body, and I will eat only when I am hungry."

"From now on, I will listen to my body, and I will eat only when I am hungry."

Are you still hungry? If so, take another bite, and chew it slowly. If not, wait to take a bite until after you have gone through the next section.

From now on, you will eat only when you are hungry, and you will lose weight.

Say to yourself, silently or out loud:

"From now on, I will eat only when I am hungry, and I will lose weight."

Say it three more times:

"From now on, I will eat only when I am hungry, and I will lose weight."

"From now on, I will eat only when I am hungry, and I will lose weight."

> **"From now on, I will eat only when I am hungry, and I will lose weight."**

Are you still hungry? If so, take another bite, and chew it slowly. If not, wait to take a bite until after you have gone through the next section.

Be patient. You will lose weight.

Say to yourself, silently or out loud:

> **"I will be patient. I will lose weight."**

Say it three more times:

> **"I will be patient. I will lose weight."**

> **"I will be patient. I will lose weight."**

> **"I will be patient. I will lose weight."**

This concludes the pacing program. If you would like to continue eating, return to any point in the pacing program and resume reading.

* This script is copyright © by ACOR Programs, Inc. ACOR Programs, Inc. grants individuals the right to record the material for personal use only. All commercial uses are strictly forbidden. The full script is available in both audio and video formats; see page 326-327 for ordering information.

DAY 3

Assignment

1. Decrease fat in your diet so it accounts for less than 20 percent of your total calories for the day. To accomplish this, increase your intake of foods that have 10 percent or less of their calories from fat and cut back significantly on foods with 30 percent or more of their calories from fat.

2. Cover 1,500 feet (walking or running at any pace, continuously or in smaller segments).

3. Walk up one flight of stairs.

4. Eat your meals using the pacing system, pausing 30 seconds between each bite.

5. Eat at least three meals.

6. Choose one of the following:

    a. Make a pleasant change in the way you eat a meal. Set an especially pretty table with flowers or candles, or use your best dishes to turn an ordinary lunch or dinner into a special occasion.

    b. Serve yourself a meal today using a smaller plate.

7. Using your Self-Monitoring tearout chart, score yourself at the end of the day for goals accomplished.

DAY 4

SHOPPING

Making the Best Use of Food Labels

In 1994, the Food and Drug Administration began requiring food manufacturers to display new nutritional labels on most foods. These "Nutritional Facts" labels make the fat content of foods and other information very accessible.

The three most important items on the food label as far as losing weight is concerned are: *Serving Size, Calories,* and *Calories from Fat.*

Serving Size. Most of us have our own idea of what constitutes a "serving." For some people, a serving of chicken means a boneless breast; for others, it's a breast, a thigh, a wing, and a leg. For some, a serving of pasta is just enough to cover a small plate; for others, it's a pile of spaghetti four inches high that spans a large dish.

Unfortunately, our ideas about serving size rarely match up with the ones that food manufacturers list on nutritional labels. In most cases, our servings are much more generous. Pasta is one of the best examples of this discrepancy. Although the manufacturer insists there are eight servings in each box of spaghetti, my wife and I routinely cook half the box for the two of us. Bagels are another good example. Did you know that one bagel is considered *two* servings?

Manufacturers are purposely stingy with their portion sizes to make it look like you're getting more for your money. You might not buy a $4 box of breakfast cereal that says it contains only four servings. When it claims to contain ten, it seems like a bargain. Decreasing the serving size also makes the product look more appealing from a nutritional standpoint. A smaller serving size automatically contains less calories and less fat than a larger one.

Regardless of what the label says, a serving size is the amount you choose to put on your plate. So, even if you are choosing low-fat or nonfat foods, you can totally undermine your efforts by overloading on them. Pretzels are a good example. Pretzels are considered a low-fat snack, because most pretzels get only 10 to 20 percent of their calories from fat. One ounce of almost any pretzel (that's the official serving size) contains 110 calories. But who eats just one ounce? The average person would consider two or three ounces a "normal" serving—still a relatively small amount of food, but between 220 and 330 calories worth of energy. That's a lot of calories for a low-fat snack. By the way, things are no better when you switch to fat-free pretzels, which contain the same 110 calories per ounce. They may be healthier calories, because they are not coming from fat, but they'll still add pounds to your body if they push your total caloric intake for the day over the amount you burn.

Serving sizes can get you into trouble with cereals, too. There are many wonderful low-fat cereals available today, but—in my opinion—the manufacturers' serving sizes are completely unrealistic. The average serving size of one ounce often translates into only half a cup of cereal. I can't remember the last time I stopped at half a cup, and I'm not that different from other cereal eaters. Again, even the fat-free brands can get you into trouble if you're not mindful of serving sizes. The extra calories you consume by eating two ounces instead of one (about 100) won't affect your weight significantly unless you're a regular cereal eater and you repeat the action five or six times a week, all year long. If you do that, you've just packed ten extra pounds of weight onto your frame.

Perhaps the worst culprits when it comes to serving sizes are the companies pushing those new nonfat cookies. The label says that one serving equals 13 cookies—which sounds like a lot. But those cookies are so small, many people go far beyond the allotted 13 before they are satisfied.

So, what's my advice? Read labels before you buy any food, and take a careful look at the manufacturer's portion size. Don't let yourself be tricked into buying foods that will end up stuffing you with more calories than the choices you used to make. And if you're going to eat loads of nonfat cookie calories because you can't stop with just one or two servings, look for a better snack alternative.

What else can you do if your serving size is larger than theirs? Start with theirs (for example, pour only one of the manufacturer's cereal portions into your bowl). If you still want more after you've finished that portion, go ahead and pour another one—but wait until you've eaten the first to make that decision. Also, slow your eating pace even more than usual. You'll be surprised how

THE NEW FOOD-LABEL TERMINOLOGY

Federal regulations have standardized the meaning of key words that often appear on food packaging. The FDA has prescribed the definitions listed here for the following terms:

FAT-FREE   Less than 0.5 grams of fat per serving. These are the foods you should increase most dramatically in your diet.

LOW-FAT   Three grams or less of fat per serving. You can usually eat these foods without concern, unless you eat several servings.

LEAN   Less than ten grams of fat, four grams of saturated fat, and 95 milligrams of cholesterol per serving. You need to be careful with these foods and read the rest of the label carefully, since they can contain as many as 89 fat calories per serving.

LIGHT (LITE)   One-third fewer calories, or no more than one-half the fat of the higher calorie, higher fat version. These foods are potentially risky; if you're consuming "light" granola that has one-half the fat of the higher-fat granola, you'll still be eating lots of fat.

CHOLESTEROL-FREE   Less than two milligrams of cholesterol and two grams (or less) of saturated fat per serving. The risk here is that the food contains lots of unsaturated fat (perhaps vegetable oils), which will contribute to your overall fat intake.

much larger the manufacturer's serving size will seem when you eat it more slowly. If that sounds silly, just try it once. I think you'll change your mind.

Calories. Although calories aren't as important to this weight-loss program as fat, it's very useful to know the number of calories contained in the given serving size. Generally, you're better off selecting foods that have a low number of calories and a large serving size; they'll be low in fat as well.

Calories from Fat. As the name indicates, these are the actual number of fat calories in each serving size. This figure includes all types of fat (saturated, monounsaturated, polyunsaturated).

You can use the numbers listed for *Calories* and *Calories from Fat* to determine the percentage of calories from fat in a given serving. Here's how to make this calculation:

- Divide the number of *Calories from Fat* by the total *Calories* in the serving size.

- Take the result, and multiply it by 100 to change it to a percentage. (The fastest way to do this is to move the decimal point two digits to the right.) This figure is the *percentage of calories that comes from fat.*

For example, using the sample label on this page, you would divide 30 (the number of *Calories from Fat*) by 90 (the number of *Calories* in a serving), arriving at a result of .33.

Nutrition Facts	
Serving Size ½ cup (114g)	
Servings Per Container 4	

Amount Per Serving	
Calories 90	Calories from Fat 30

	% Daily Value*
Total Fat 3g	5%
Saturated Fat 0g	0%
Cholesterol 0mg	0%
Sodium 300mg	13%
Total Carbohydrate 13g	4%
Dietary Fiber 3g	12%
Sugars 3g	
Protein 3g	

Vitamin A	80%	•	Vitamin C	60%
Calcium	4%	•	Iron	4%

* Percent Daily Values are based on a 2,000 calorie diet. Your daily values may be higher or lower depending on your calorie needs:

		Calories	2,000	2,500
Total Fat	Less than		65g	80g
Sat Fat	Less than		20g	25g
Cholesterol	Less than		300mg	300mg
Sodium	Less than		2,400mg	2,400mg
Total Carbohydrate			300g	375g
Fiber			25g	30g

Calories per gram:
Fat 9 • Carbohydrate 4 • Protein 4

Then multiply that figure by 100, converting it to 33 percent. In this example, this particular food would not be encouraged on our weight-loss program (or it would have to be eaten very sparingly) because of the high percentage of its calories that comes from fat.

Here is something else you will find on the food label:

Total Fat (in grams). When you're comparison shopping, the lower the total fat content, the better. Below the *Total Fat* listing, you will find a breakdown of *Saturated Fat*, which is particularly important if you are trying to control your cholesterol level; however, when it comes to losing weight, *all* types of fat are important, not just saturated.

The remainder of the label contains valuable information about the content of cholesterol, sodium, total carbohydrate (including dietary fiber and sugars), protein, and certain vitamins and minerals (such as vitamins A and C, calcium and iron). While it's useful for you to become familiar with the amounts of these nutrients in a particular food product, it is the fat content that will make the difference when you're trying to control your weight.

There is one problem with the new nutrition label: The FDA has created confusion by assigning each label listing a "Percent Daily Value" (see the right-hand column of the sample label, page 128). Because all these percentages are based on a 2,000-calorie diet, if you're consuming less than that in order to lose weight, the percentages will not be accurate for you. I suggest that you ignore these percentages, and concentrate instead on the three key elements for weight loss: *Serving Size, Calories,* and *Calories from Fat.* The only exception to this guideline relates to Total Fat; if you want to keep track of the amount of fat (in grams) that you're consuming, the *Total Fat* listing can be useful.

High-Fat Foods

In this weight-loss plan, you need to avoid or drastically minimize your consumption of all foods that derive 30 percent or more of their calories from fat. A complete list of these foods could go on for dozens of pages; here is just a sampling of the categories of fat-rich foods in the American diet. By reading food labels carefully, you'll discover for yourself the foods that don't belong in your supermarket shopping cart.

MEAT AND FISH

You do not need to eliminate meat from your diet completely. But—because meat is high in total fat, saturated fat, and dietary cholesterol—you should cut back on the amount of meat you consume. Choose the cuts that are lowest in fat, and limit portion sizes. Neither of these actions is as difficult as you may think.

In recent years, meat producers have adopted new breeding and feeding methods that have reduced the fat content of their animals. Even so, beef is still a major source of fat in the American diet. In general, you should eat beef less frequently, and even then only with care. When choosing beef, concentrate on cuts that have the least amount of visible fat or marbling throughout the muscle. Also keep in mind that even when beef appears lean, it still has lots of fat. As the table "Fat Content of Common Meat and Fish" on page 131 shows, cuts such as tip round, top round, and top sirloin have less fat than other cuts. Avoid the fattiest cuts, which include ribs and tenderloin. Look for low-fat grades of ground beef, too. And stay away from liver, kidney, heart, and tongue, except on rare occasions.

Keep your portion sizes small as well. I recommend about three or four ounces per serving. That's a piece approximately the size of a deck of playing cards. You can further cut the amount of fat in each serving of meat by extending these dishes with beans, pasta, grains, and vegetables that are low in fat. Try adding rice, barley, potatoes, or carrots to a meat recipe; you won't lose much of the robust meat flavor that you may enjoy, but you will lose some of meat's potential to add pounds to your waistline.

In many (though certainly not all) instances, you are better off choosing poultry or fish than beef. Depending on the type you choose, poultry or fish can be lower in total fat. For instance, in seafood, fat levels are especially low in cod, haddock, and yellow-

FAT CONTENT OF COMMON MEAT AND FISH

	Portion	Total Fat (grams)	% Fat Calories
Bass, freshwater, broiled	3 oz.	4.0	29%
Beef, eye of round, lean, trimmed, roasted	3 oz.	3.0	20%
Beef rib, small end, lean, trimmed, broiled	3 oz.	7.4	40%
Beef tenderloin, lean, trimmed, broiled	3 oz.	7.5	40%
Beef, tip round, lean, trimmed, roasted	3 oz.	4.5	28%
Beef, top round, lean, trimmed, braised	3 oz.	3.4	19%
Beef top sirloin, lean trimmed, broiled	3 oz.	4.8	28%
Chicken breast, with skin, roasted	3 oz.	6.6	36%
Chicken breast, without skin, roasted	3 oz.	3.1	20%
Chicken, dark meat, without skin, roasted	3 oz.	8.3	43%
Chicken, white meat, without skin, roasted	3 oz.	3.8	23%
Cod, Atlantic, broiled	3 oz.	0.7	7%
Ground beef, 7% fat, by weight, broiled or baked	3 oz.	7.0	42%
Haddock, broiled	3 oz.	0.8	8%
Halibut, broiled	3 oz.	2.5	19%
Salmon, pink, broiled	3 oz.	3.8	27%
Tuna, yellowfin, fresh, broiled	3 oz.	1.0	8%
Turkey, dark meat, without skin, roasted	3 oz.	6.1	35%
Turkey, light meat, without skin, roasted	3 oz.	2.7	18%

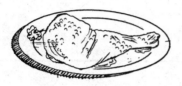

CHICKEN WITH SKIN

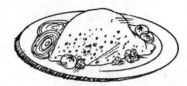

**CHICKEN BREAST
WITHOUT SKIN**

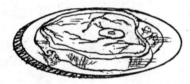

FATTY CUT OF BEEF

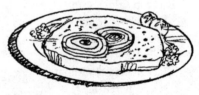

LEAN CUT OF BEEF

You can decrease the amount of fat you eat by making wise choices of meat in your diet. As the examples above show, you can cut your fat intake by switching from dark chicken with skin to chicken breast without skin; and by giving up fatty cuts of beef in favor of leaner cuts.

fin tuna. Types of seafood that are higher in fat include bass, herring, and sardines. Cooked freshwater bass, for instance, contains four grams of total fat in a three-ounce serving, so that about 29 percent of its calories come from fat. Compare those numbers to those for the same size serving of haddock, which contains less than one gram of fat and gets about 8 percent of its calories from fat.

When choosing chicken and turkey, bear in mind that light meat contains less fat than dark meat. If you choose dark meat, you may not be any better off than you would be if you ate beef instead. For instance, while skinless dark chicken meat contains 8.3 grams of total fat in a typical three-ounce cooked serving (43 percent of calories from fat), skinless light meat contains much less: 3.8 grams (23 percent of calories from fat). Removing the skin before eating, incidentally, can make a big difference in the fat content; if you leave the skin on that serving of light chicken meat, the percentage of calories from fat nearly doubles.

One other note about poultry: Ground chicken or turkey may not be as low in fat as you think, unless you have it ground to order. Manufacturers of commercially ground poultry are permitted to grind some skin in with the rest of the chicken or turkey, significantly raising the percentage of calories from fat. You might consider grinding skinless turkey breast in your own meat grinder so that you keep the fat content right where it belongs.

DAIRY PRODUCTS

Dairy products are important and economical sources of calcium, protein, and vitamin D. However, if you don't select the right products, this food category can also become a very troublesome source of excess fat. For example, you need to choose cheese carefully and eat it in smaller amounts than you might be used to.

Although whole milk and low-fat milk are 3.3 percent and 2 percent fat by weight, those numbers are actually quite misleading, because milk is mostly water. When you calculate the actual number of calories in milk that comes from fat, the figures are unsettling. In whole milk (total calories: 150 per eight-ounce glass), 49 percent of the calories are fat calories; that figure drops (but not by much) to 37 percent for 2 percent milk (total calories: 121 per glass). You're much better off choosing "nonfat" or skim milk, which gets only about 4 percent of its calories from fat (total calories: 86 per glass).

Cheese tends to be brimming with fat; in most cheeses, 65 to 75 percent of the calories come from fat. Even the "low-fat" or "part-skim" cheeses contain more fat than you might think. For example, part-skim ricotta, although lower in fat than the whole milk variety, still has a fat content equal to 51 percent of its calo-

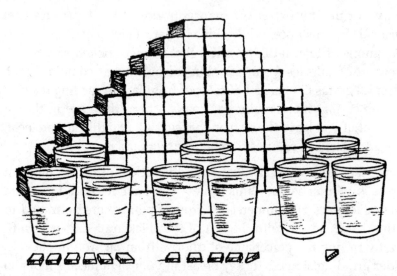

Making the switch from whole milk to nonfat milk can significantly reduce your fat intake. If you were to drink three glasses of whole milk a day for a year, you'd consume fat equal to the amount in 88 sticks of butter. On a daily basis, drinking three glasses of whole milk would be equivalent to consuming six pats of butter, compared to 4½ pats with low-fat milk and ½ pat with non-fat.

ries. Some "fat-free" varieties of cheese have recently become available, and although their flavor and texture may not be as good as the real thing, many people have adapted well to them, and use them in salads and sauces. Other individuals, however, still find such cheeses difficult to stomach, and opt for the low-fat choices instead.

Since you can choose so many other dairy foods that are low in fat, and since most cheeses (except the fat-free varieties) are way over our 30 percent fat guideline, if you love cheese, I suggest treating it as a delicacy. That means eating cheese less often and in much smaller portions, and trying to stick with the low-fat alternatives. Limit your portion sizes to about one-third what you would have eaten in the past. Another way to beat the fat trap is to grate Parmesan, cheddar, or sapsago cheese, and sprinkle it on casseroles or main dishes; you'll be able to enjoy the flavor of cheese without sabotaging your fat-lowering efforts.

Many lower-fat dairy alternatives are now available in your supermarket, including fat-free frozen dairy desserts and nonfat yogurt,

FAT CONTENT OF COMMON DAIRY PRODUCTS

	Portion	Total Fat (grams)	% Fat Calories
American cheese, fat-free singles	1 oz.	0	0%
Butter	1 Tbs. or 3 pats	12.2	100%
Cheddar cheese, mild or sharp	1 oz.	2.0	36%
Cottage cheese, 1% fat	.5 cup	1.2	13%
Cottage cheese, 2% fat	.5 cup	2.2	20%
Cream, coffee	1 Tbs.	2.9	90%
Milk, evaporated skim, canned	.5 cup	0.3	3%
Milk, skim or nonfat	1 cup	0.4	4%
Milk, 1% fat	1 cup	2.6	23%
Milk, 2% fat	1 cup	5.0	37%
Milk, whole	1 cup	8.2	49%
Mozzarella cheese, reduced fat	1 oz.	3.0	39%
Mozzarella cheese, fat-free	1 oz.	0	0%
Ricotta cheese, part skim	1 oz.	2.2	51%
Sour cream, reduced fat	1 oz.	3.0	68%
Swiss cheese	1 oz.	7.8	66%
Yogurt, 1% milkfat, fruit on bottom	8 oz.	3.0	11%
Yogurt, nonfat, vanilla	8 oz.	0	0%

which can be used as a substitute for sour cream in recipes. (A cup of plain nonfat yogurt has no fat, while an equal amount of regular sour cream contains about 42 grams or nearly 400 fat calories!) You can also eliminate a lot of fat by using nonfat yogurt as a salad dressing or as a topping for baked potatoes.

As for butter and margarine, they will cost you dearly in terms of fat content. All of butter's calories come from fat. And don't expect to fare any better with margarine, because 100 percent of its calories are derived from fat, too. You can cut back on the fat a little by selecting reduced-calorie or diet varieties of margarine.

Since they are diluted with water, tablespoon for tablespoon they have as little as half the fat (and half the calories) of regular margarine. But their percentage of fat is still far above the 30 percent limit we've established for most foods in this eating plan, so you really ought to use jam or jelly on your morning toast instead. If you absolutely can't bear the thought of giving up butter or margarine completely, save it for special occasions, and then cut your portion size to one-third of what you once used. You'll still get the feel and flavor, but without all those extra fat calories. (See "Fat Content of Common Dairy Products," page 135.)

OILS

When heart disease is the concern, some oils are better than others. When weight loss is your goal, however, all oils should be treated identically—by avoiding or drastically reducing your intake of them. They are all 100 percent fat.

Food manufacturers are making it very easy to cut back on fat from one source: salad dressings. Fat-free dressings have become widely available, and contain no fat, no cholesterol, and relatively few calories. If you are using a higher-fat dressing, however, in which more than 30 percent of calories come from fat, you need to use much less of it—about one-third of what you once used.

FAT CONTENT OF COMMON OILS AND SPREADS

	Portion	Total Fat (grams)	% Fat Calories
Canola oil	1 Tbs.	13.6	100%
Margarine, regular, soft	1 Tbs.	11.0	100%
Margarine, whipped	1 Tbs.	7.0	90%
Margarine, soft, reduced calorie	1 Tbs.	6.0	84%
Margarine, soft, extra light spread, tub	1 Tbs.	4.0	80%
Mayonnaise, cholesterol free, reduced calorie	1 Tbs.	5.0	90%
Mayonnaise, dressing, non-fat	1 Tbs.	0	0%
Olive oil	1 Tbs.	13.5	100%
Safflower oil	1 Tbs.	13.6	100%

SNACKS AND DESSERTS

As with salad dressings, snacks and desserts need not undermine your low-fat dietary program. Your supermarket carries dozens of low-fat and nonfat snack foods and desserts; even some cookies and cakes qualify. Some premium ice creams now come in fat-free varieties, containing zero fat and zero cholesterol in flavors as irresistible as chocolate fudge. Most commercial ice cream and yogurt shops now offer nonfat versions of their desserts, too, but you still need to be careful with your portion sizes.

Let's not forget about the wonderful desserts and snacks that nature created for us. Frankly, if you're looking for a very low-fat treat, you can't do any better than to select a tasty fruit. Or you can air-pop some popcorn, sprinkling it with a little Parmesan cheese or herbs or spices for flavor. (See "Fat Content of Common Snacks and Desserts" below.)

FAT CONTENT OF COMMON SNACKS AND DESSERTS

	Portion	Total Fat (grams)	% Fat Calories
Applesauce, unsweetened	.5 cup	0.1	2%
Dairy dessert, nonfat	.5 cup	0	0%
Popcorn, microwavable, light, butter-flavored	3 cups	2.0	30%
Popcorn, popped without fat, salted	3 cups	1.2	12%
Sherbet	.5 cup	1.0	8%
Strawberries, fresh	.5 cup	0.3	12%
Yogurt, frozen, low-fat	3 fluid oz.	1.0	7%
Yogurt, frozen, nonfat	3 fluid oz.	0	0%

The Percentage Paradox

The percentage system we have created in this book—increasing your intake of foods with 10 percent or less of their calories from fat, and cutting back drastically on foods with 30 percent or more of their calories from fat—works extremely well in most instances. By choosing foods with low-fat percentages, you'll automatically be selecting foods that are low in calories, too. Broccoli, for example, derives 9 percent of its calories from fat, and contains only 12 calories in a half-cup serving (yes, vegetables like broccoli do actually contain fat, but this fat is almost insignificant within the context of a low-fat diet).

However, some foods, particularly snack foods, present a paradox that runs counter to this basic tenet of our program. Even if they have relatively modest fat percentages—or in some cases, contain no fat at all—they can be high in calories ("calorically dense"). One Bavarian-style pretzel, for instance, contains absolutely no fat—but it still has as many as 100 calories (that's a lot of calories when you consider that few of us stop eating after just one pretzel!).

Pickles are another good example of this paradox—but in this case, pickles are still a good choice for our program. About 24 percent of a pickle's calories come from fat, which generally means that it can be incorporated into your diet in a thoughtful and careful manner. But when you look at the number of calories in an average pickle, you'll find only three calories! Thus, pickles can be eaten much more freely than most other foods with 24 percent fat calories.

So even though the "percentage of calories from fat" is a useful guideline for nearly all foods, it can be misleading in some cases. To identify the caloric density of foods, read nutrition labels carefully. Look at the number of calories in an official serving size, then think about how many of these "servings" you're likely to eat. If you really can stop with one occasional pretzel, the 100 calories won't pose an obstacle to your weight-loss efforts; but one pretzel every day will put ten pounds on your body by the end of the year! If you sense you're going to eat four of them at a sitting, count to ten instead and find a better alternative.

DAY 4

Assignment

1. Decrease fat in your diet so it accounts for less than 20 percent of your total calories for the day. To accomplish this, increase your intake of foods that have 10 percent or less of their calories from fat and cut back significantly on foods with 30 percent or more of their calories from fat.

2. Cover 2,000 feet (walking or running at any pace, continuously or in smaller segments).

3. Walk up one flight of stairs.

4. Eat your meals using the pacing system, pausing 30 seconds between each bite.

5. Eat at least three meals.

6. Choose one of the following:

   a. Read the labels on at least five foods in your kitchen. Make a list of those with a caloric fat content over 30 percent and find replacements for them the next time you go shopping.

   b. Take a look at your herbs and spices. When you're cutting down on fat, herbs and spices can add new and exciting flavors to replace the fat. Make a list of herbs and spices to buy next time you're shopping. Oregano, garlic or garlic powder, dill, and basil are just a few of the most versatile.

7. Using your Self-Monitoring tearout chart, score yourself at the end of the day for goals accomplished.

DAY 5

EXERCISE HINTS

Estimating Distances

As you have already discovered, our program includes some pretty specific exercise assignments. On the first day, for example, you were asked to climb one flight of stairs and walk 500 feet. This is what people told us they wanted in an exercise program. So we were surprised some of them then began to ask: "How far is 500 feet?"

In a moment, I'll show you several ways for measuring the distance of your walks, but first let me say the following: Stop worrying about precise distances. Just get out there and have a little fun. So what if you are 50 feet short today and 100 feet long tomorrow? Start walking, and the distance will take care of itself. Now, if you feel you still need more structure, here's how to measure the distance of your workouts.

The easiest way to determine how far you're walking is to get in your car and "clock" your route. Reset your car's odometer to zero, then drive your usual walking route. (If you have more than one route, drive them all.) Pull over every half mile and identify a landmark you can easily recognize when you're covering the route on foot. Write down the landmarks and distances from home (or wherever your route starts) so you can learn them later, or carry the "route map" with you on your walks. Before long, you won't need the map. You'll quickly be able to judge distances by "feel."

If you don't drive, or you walk a route that cannot be driven, you can still use landmarks to monitor your progress. For example, you can determine the average lot size in your neighborhood, and then count houses as you walk. If lots in your neighborhood are 100 feet wide, you'll cover one mile every 53 houses. If your walking route has evenly spaced phone poles, calculate the distance

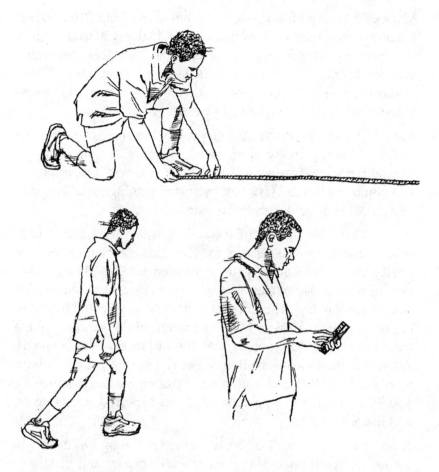

To determine the distances you walk, first measure how much ground you cover with each stride at your normal walking speed. Then count the number of steps you take when walking particular routes, and multiply that number by the length of your stride. The result is the distance you're walking on that particular route.

between poles and then count poles as you walk. Some people find the counting very relaxing (it takes their mind off everything else); others find it tedious. Give it a try to see how it works for you.

Another way to measure the distance you're covering is to count the number of steps you've taken. But first, you've got to know your "stride length," or how much ground you cover with each step.

Here's a simple way to measure your stride length:

Mark off a known distance—ranging anywhere from 20 to 100 feet in length—and then see how many steps it takes you to cover that distance at your normal exercise pace. You can then determine your stride length by dividing the distance by the number of steps it took to cover it. For example, if you covered 25 feet in ten steps, your stride length is two and a half feet.

Keep in mind that the length of your stride changes with your speed. As you increase your speed, your legs begin to hit the ground farther and farther apart. So, as your fitness level improves and you begin to walk faster (or even start jogging), you'll need to recalculate your stride length from time to time.

If you use the "stride length" method, consider purchasing a pedometer to measure the distance for you. This is a motion-sensitive device that you wear on your waistband while walking (some people wear a pedometer all day long to measure their overall activity for the day). The simplest pedometers just count the number of steps you've taken (you then multiply this number by the length of your stride to determine the distance you've covered). Electronic models are available that can be programmed with your stride length, and automatically calculate the distance for you. Pedometers can be purchased at most sporting goods stores, and cost $10 to $25.

After you've been walking for a while, estimating distances will get easier. You'll establish a regular walking pace and be able to determine how far you've gone based upon the amount of time you walk. (For instance, I walk briskly, covering about four and a half miles in an hour. When I walk for 30 minutes, I can be pretty sure I've covered two and a quarter miles.)

EXERCISE EQUIVALENTS

The exercise program you are using during the first 28 days is built around two "required" assignments—walking and stair climbing. We have selected these two activities because they are easy to do, safe, require no special training or expensive equipment, can be done by people of any age, allow plenty of room for "growth," and meet the basic goals of this program (they burn fat and preserve muscle mass). However, there is no reason you can't substitute other types of exercise for both activities, as long as they are fairly equivalent with respect to the results they produce. In fact, I encourage you to choose the activities you enjoy most. If you don't like to walk, but love to swim, for example, don't force yourself to complete the walking assignments. If you do, chances are you'll be unhappy and give up on the exercise completely.

Choose the type of exercises you enjoy doing and develop a program similar to the one we've devised for walking. Here are a few guidelines to help you:

- **Select activities that will enable you to burn as many calories as you would walking.** Use the calorie chart provided on page 95 to determine how the alternative activities you choose compare to walking. For example: Brisk walking burns about six calories per minute; swimming burns about one and a half times that amount (nine calories per minute). Since walking 500 feet would take you about two minutes, if you plan to swim you would have to do it for only one minute and twenty seconds your first day and add that same amount of time every day thereafter.

- **Choose activities that will strengthen and tone the muscles of your lower body.** Both walking and stair climbing strengthen the muscles of your legs and buttocks and help protect you against muscle loss as you lose weight. Select alternative activities that also work these muscle groups (cycling, roller blading, and step aerobics are good examples), or add a series of leg lifts and squats to your workout regimen.

- **Choose activities that will improve your level of aerobic conditioning.** Consider activities like swimming, aerobic dancing, cycling, and jumping rope. Monitor your pulse rate during exercise sessions to ensure that the intensity of your activity is sufficient to improve your fitness level. For example, if you pedal too slowly, cycling may not raise your heart rate as much as walking.

WALKING FOR YOUR HEART

After a few weeks of regular walking, you'll probably find that even though you're walking farther, the walking itself is getting easier. That's because your body is becoming aerobically conditioned. Your heart muscle is getting stronger and pumping blood more efficiently. As a result, more blood is delivered with each heartbeat, so your heart can beat more slowly and still supply enough blood to your body. Because of this conditioning process, your heart rate will not speed up as much as it did when you first started exercising, and your breathing will be easier and more regular.

As your physical condition continues to improve, walking will undoubtedly become more comfortable and more pleasant. This is a signal to push yourself a bit harder and increase your walking speed. Although walking a given distance slowly burns up as many calories as walking it quickly, increasing your pace offers you an additional benefit: It further improves your level of aerobic fitness. To build aerobic conditioning you should strive to keep your heart rate between 50 and 70 percent of its maximum (see page 92 for information about how to estimate your maximum heart rate). Increasing your speed is the simplest way to bring your heart rate back up after conditioning has allowed it to drop below the target zone. But, increases should be made gradually and carefully to avoid overexerting yourself and raising your heart rate too high. Here's a safe way to do it:

At regular intervals (perhaps weekly), check to see if your heart rate has fallen below your target zone. Five or ten minutes into your walk, stop and measure your pulse. Place your index and middle fingers over the artery in your wrist (see diagram). Count the number of beats, or "pulses," you feel in 30 seconds. Multiply this number by two to determine the number of times your heart is beating each minute.

If your heart rate is below 50 percent of its maximum, increase your walking speed slightly and measure your pulse again after five minutes. If the faster pace raises your heart rate back up in the target zone, complete your walk at this new speed. If your

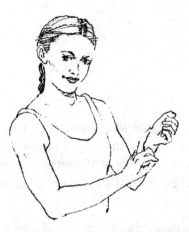

Several minutes into your walk, stop momentarily to measure your pulse. With your index and middle fingers placed over the artery in your wrist, count the number of beats in 30 seconds, and then multiply by two to calculate the number of beats in a minute. Use this information to determine if you are within your target zone.

heart rate is still too low, increase your speed a little more and recheck your pulse a few minutes later.

Another way to get your heart rate back up into the target zone is to choose a more challenging walking route. If you're used to walking a very flat route, pick a new one that has a few small hills. Once you can climb them with ease, find routes with even steeper or longer inclines. In addition to improving your aerobic condition, walking hillier routes will help you maintain and strengthen the muscles of your lower body in a way that flat walking can't.

DAY 5

Assignment

1. Decrease fat in your diet so it accounts for less than 20 percent of your total calories for the day. To accomplish this, increase your intake of foods that have 10 percent or less of their calories from fat and cut back significantly on foods with 30 percent or more of their calories from fat.

2. Cover 2,500 feet (walking or running at any pace, continuously or in smaller segments).

3. Walk up one flight of stairs.

4. Eat your meals using the pacing system, pausing 30 seconds between each bite.

5. Eat at least three meals.

6. Choose one of the following:

   a. Take a good look at your walking shoes. Make sure they fit well and offer you good support. If not, buy a new pair that meets the requirements of your walking regimen. Stores that sell athletic shoes often carry a line of shoes made specifically for walking. Many people find these specially designed walking shoes so comfortable, they wear them all the time.

   b. Next time you park your car in a parking lot, choose the space farthest from your destination instead of the closest one.

7. Using your Self-Monitoring tearout chart, score yourself at the end of the day for goals accomplished.

DAY 6

THINKING SMALL FOR BIG RESULTS

Since you started this program, you've probably had a goal in mind of the amount of weight you want to lose. But whether your target is 10, 30, or 100 pounds, your chances of success are much greater if you work at it in tiny increments. Thinking small, in fact, is a way to lose big.

Steady, predictable declines in weight, no matter how small, will eventually get you to your goal, since they can add up to significant losses over long periods of time.

In this program, I want you to set a goal of losing just three ounces of body fat a day. That's all—just three ounces. It certainly doesn't sound like much, does it? But three ounces a day over many weeks and months translate into large amounts of lost weight. By losing just three ounces a day (the equivalent of about 660 calories), your weight will decline one pound, five ounces a week—or 68 pounds over the course of a year! Even if you have 100 pounds to lose, it's important to do it in this slow, steady manner, following our guidelines so you lose body fat, not lean tissue.

The way this program has been set up, you are probably already on course to lose those three ounces a day. In fact, this three-ounce target is just another way of looking at what you've already begun doing. Each of the following three strategies will produce a weight decline of one ounce:

- Lose one ounce a day by cutting the fat in your diet. Find 220 calories of fat a day that you can eliminate.

- Lose one ounce a day by leaving a little food (220 calories worth) on your plate, or making your serving sizes a little smaller. Make it easy on yourself, and leave that extra food on the serving trays—or in the kitchen.

- Lose one ounce a day through exercise, burning off 220 calories.

It really won't take much to reach each of these three goals every day. For example, to help reduce your fat intake by 220 calories a day, you could:

- Cut 2 tablespoons of butter from your diet, and save 200 calories.

- Eliminate 2 tablespoons of oil, and save 240 calories.

- Switch from whole milk to skim milk, and in drinking 3 cups a day, consume 195 fewer calories.

Leaving small amounts of food on your plate can make a big difference, too:

- Don't eat one-third of a typical frozen dinner, and save 125 calories.

- Leave one-half of a slice of chocolate cake, and save 150 calories.

- Don't eat one-third of a typical serving of bacon and eggs, and save 100 calories.

To help achieve your goal of losing an ounce (220 calories) during exercise, you could:

- Walk three miles in an hour, and burn 240 calories (in a 150-pound person).

- Garden for 30 minutes, and lose from 120 to 270 calories.

- Do housework for 45 minutes, and burn 150 calories.

Stay concentrated on *three ounces a day*. Again, if you try to speed up your weight loss, you may end up destroying muscle, not losing body fat. So to protect your lean tissue, aim for this steady, three-ounce-a-day pace. If you maintain it consistently—day in, day out—you'll lose 68 pounds a year. That's a very realistic goal, and it will allow you to lose as much weight as you want.

DAY 6

Assignment

1. Decrease fat in your diet so it accounts for less than 20 percent of your total calories for the day. To accomplish this, increase your intake of foods that have 10 percent or less of their calories from fat and cut back significantly on foods with 30 percent or more of their calories from fat.

2. Cover 3,000 feet (walking or running at any pace, continuously or in smaller segments).

3. Walk up one flight of stairs.

4. Eat your meals using the pacing system, pausing 30 seconds between each bite.

5. Eat at least three meals.

6. Choose one of the following:

   a. Transform a favorite high-fat recipe into a low-fat version. For example, if your recipe calls for frying, broil; if the recipe calls for sautéeing in oil or butter, use defatted chicken broth and non-stick cookware.

   b. Lose an ounce today through a little extra activity: Ride your bicycle for 30 minutes; take your dog for an extra walk; play a round of golf.

7. Using your Self-Monitoring tearout chart, score yourself at the end of the day for goals accomplished.

DAY 7

REACTIVE EATING
AND HOW TO OVERCOME IT

In the animal kingdom, obesity rarely occurs in the wild. Yet our pampered house pets—fed on a human schedule that has nothing to do with biological need—often become fat. We don't know how common obesity was for primitive humans, but in modern men and women it is rampant, and the human feeding schedule probably plays a significant role. Throughout history, humans have used food as a social and emotional tool, attaching it to celebration, social gatherings, and familial bonding.

In spite of these social and emotional attachments to food, and its plentiful availability, some people are able to turn aside temptation and eat only when they feel truly hungry. I call these people biologic eaters. They may eat a lot when they sit down to a meal, but they almost never eat just because food is available. In fact, some biologic eaters, if they are not hungry, turn down even their favorite foods. They leave the table with food still on their plates. On their birthday, they eat one piece of cake and put the rest away. These people are almost always normal weight.

Biologic Versus Reactive Eating

Many of us would eat several pieces of that birthday cake, compelled by forces that have nothing to do with hunger or social custom. I call this kind of eating "reactive eating." We are rushed, so we eat whatever is available whenever we have time. We are stressed, and we eat because food makes us feel better. And for those of us who associate food with love and nurturing, eating can provide a sense of comfort, or replicate a positive feeling from childhood that is missing from our present lives. If our parents used food as a reward, we may overeat as adults in order to feel good about ourselves.

Eating can also be a means of gaining control. During childhood, overeating or undereating is a way we can control others, to get attention or to punish our parents for hurting or neglecting us. Eating may also be a way of asserting control over our own bodies. Some people have difficulty giving up obesity—on a subconscious level, if not a conscious one—because being overweight serves some function in their lives. Obesity may provide a protective shield, keeping people away so we don't have to deal with closeness or uncomfortable social situations. A weight problem may also serve as a defense mechanism, an excuse for social failure and distant relationships, especially with parents. In men, being big may actually be seen as an advantage: a symbol of power, strength, and a capacity to intimidate.

One of the most difficult aspects of dealing with reactive eating is that it very often operates at a subconscious level. Even while they are eating reactively, few people are aware of the feelings that are triggering their eating. This lack of awareness helps to explain why reliance on willpower isn't effective for losing weight and keeping it off—even among the most strong-willed people. The fact is, you can exert your will only over the behaviors you are aware of. No matter how hard you try, you cannot use your willpower to change behavior that your conscious mind doesn't recognize.

Subconscious psychological and emotional forces can interfere with your ability to override a malfunctioning weight-regulating system. In fact, at times it may almost seem as if reactive eating is your regulator's way of pushing your weight to higher levels. I'm convinced that my weight regulator works that way. So are many of the reactive eaters with whom I've spoken. Most of them were relieved to hear this theory about how the process works. For the first time, they had an explanation for their frustrating—and sometimes frightening—lack of control over their eating.

So what can you do if emotional and psychological issues are triggering you to eat when you are not biologically hungry? How do you break this vicious cycle? No single approach works for all reactive eaters. That's because reactive eaters vary enormously in their psychological and behavioral characteristics, and in the issues that trigger their reactive eating. Even in the same person, no single technique works in all situations. I've found, though, that two steps are necessary for success in controlling this eating behavior:

1. You must recognize that emotional factors are creating urges to eat when you are not biologically hungry.

2. Once you are aware that emotional and situational issues are creating urges to eat, you must consciously change your reaction to those urges so you no longer respond to them by eating.

Recognizing When Emotions Create Urges to Eat

Sometimes it's obvious that an emotional issue is triggering your eating: for example, when you gorge yourself after a fight with a loved one, after a great disappointment, or during situations of great stress. But, more often, the emotional connection goes unnoticed, and the reactive eating process operates at a subliminal level. Many reactive eaters are simply unaware how often psychological and situational triggers like stress are tempting them.

To break this pattern of reactive eating, it is essential that you increase your awareness of the connection between your eating and the psychological and situational issues that may lie behind it. Increased awareness will not necessarily make the eating urges go away, but it will help you react to them in a healthier, more appropriate manner.

Awareness enables you to make a choice. Once you're aware that emotional and situational issues are triggering your urges to eat, you can then choose to respond to the urges differently. For the first time, you can take control of the process that until now has been controlling you.

The questionnaire "Are You a Reactive Eater" on the next page will help you determine whether reactive eating is contributing to your weight problem. Even if you think you already know the answer to that question, take a moment now to respond to the questionnaire.

ARE YOU A REACTIVE EATER?

Examine your eating patterns and the feelings that pass through your mind and body before and after each meal, and ask yourself the following questions:

1. Do you eat more during times of stress? When you are sad? When you are upset?

Never   Rarely   Occasionally   Frequently   Always

2. Do thoughts of home or of family members trigger eating urges?

Never   Rarely   Occasionally   Frequently   Always

3. Are you always sabotaging your own dieting efforts?

Never   Rarely   Occasionally   Frequently   Always

4. Do you keep regaining the weight you have worked so hard to lose?

Never   Rarely   Occasionally   Frequently   Always

5. Do you weigh yourself several times a day?

Never   Rarely   Occasionally   Frequently   Always

6. Do you measure your self-worth on the scale? Do you get depressed when your weight goes up? Do you get excited when your weight goes down?

Never   Rarely   Occasionally   Frequently   Always

7. Do you eat at regular times, or at every chance you get?

Never   Rarely   Occasionally   Frequently   Always

8. Do you start snacking again right after you've eaten a meal?

Never   Rarely   Occasionally   Frequently   Always

SCORING YOUR QUESTIONNAIRE

Each *"always"* or *"frequently"* answer increases the possibility that emotional factors are triggering your eating—at least some of the time. Don't panic if two or three of your answers are *"always"* or *"frequently."* For most of us, an emotionally or situationally driven urge has triggered eating many times in our lives. But if you find yourself answering *"always"* or *"frequently"* to *most* of the questions, you've probably got a problem with emotional eating.

Do you see a pattern emerging? Are emotional and situational issues affecting your eating and interfering with your ability to override your weight-regulating system? Don't be discouraged. It's a challenge to overcome reactive eating, but it can be done.

If you are a reactive eater, you can lose weight and keep it off. But first you must understand that simply shedding pounds will not solve the underlying problem that is triggering your eating urges. If your father didn't show his love for you when you were a child, your getting thin may inspire him to compliment you now, but it will never make up for his neglect of your emotional needs then. If you are afraid to get close to people because you feel inadequate as a person, losing weight will make you thin, but won't eliminate your feelings of inadequacy. Just as no amount of food will satisfy emotional hunger, no amount of weight loss will, in itself, make you feel better about an important, unresolved emotional issue.

Sometimes, psychotherapy may be necessary to understand or treat an underlying emotional disorder. In the case of bulimia or depression, antidepressants—including a new group of drugs known as serotonin re-uptake inhibitors (Prozac, Paxil, Zoloft)—may be helpful. But for the great majority of reactive eaters, whose psychological or situational problems are far less serious, the problem can be managed through conscious, deliberate behavioral change—so you no longer react to emotional eating urges by turning to food.

Changing Your Reaction to Emotional Eating Urges

Awareness alone will not make your reactive urges to eat go away. You must literally change the way you respond to those urges, so you eat only when you are truly biologically hungry or have consciously decided to eat for another reason—for example, because you're at a social gathering or a family dinner.

How do you break a cycle that has probably gone on for most of your life? It's not easy, but one technique that many people find helpful is hunger monitoring. This technique helps you distinguish the times you are really hungry from the times when other issues are making you reach for food. Here's how hunger monitoring works.

Anytime you get an urge to take a bite of food—whether you are sitting at the dinner table, halfway through a meal, or walking through a shopping mall four hours after you last ate—ask yourself the following questions: Am I really hungry? Are these true hunger pangs I'm feeling? Or am I eating to fulfill some other need? Give yourself enough time to think about these questions. If your answers suggest that you are really hungry, take a bite of food. Then repeat the same questions to yourself before you take another bite. Repeat the sequence after every bite.

When your answers to these questions tell you that some other issue is making you think that you are hungry, you must stop and make a choice. At this point, you are no longer being driven on a subconscious level by emotional or situational stimuli that are creating urges to eat. Instead, your conscious mind is in control. Rather than expecting your willpower to be able to combat those subconscious but powerful urges, you have an opportunity to make a conscious and voluntary choice about eating.

If you think you are truly hungry, go ahead and take a bite, but chew the food slowly, taking time to savor its appearance, aroma, and taste. Enjoy the food, and relish the control that you are now exerting over your eating.

Again, bite by bite, ask yourself these questions: Am I really hungry? Are these true hunger pangs I'm feeling? Or am I eating to fulfill some other need? If the answers to those questions reveal that you are not truly hungry, it is time to walk away from the food—literally. Get up from the table and remove yourself from the food. No matter how much food is still on your plate or on the table, leave it behind.

What if you're not sure whether you're hungry or not, but you don't want to pass up the opportunity to eat if you are hungry? Then simply wait 30 seconds, and ask yourself the questions again. You are not denying yourself food, but simply delaying by 30 seconds the decision whether to eat, so you can decide on more rational grounds. You'll be surprised how much easier it is to stop your reactive eating after that 30-second delay. You'll also be amazed how much less you'll eat at every sitting.

Remember: With this technique, you can eat anything you want, anytime you are truly hungry. You can take as many bites of food as you desire, anytime you are truly hungry. You can keep eating for as long as you want, anytime you are truly hungry. If you use this technique regularly, your days of dieting and deprivation are over. So, too, are your days of reactive eating.

DAY 7

Assignment

1. Decrease fat in your diet so it accounts for less than 20 percent of your total calories for the day. To accomplish this, increase your intake of foods that have 10 percent or less of their calories from fat and cut back significantly on foods with 30 percent or more of their calories from fat.

2. Cover 3,500 feet (walking or running at any pace, continuously or in smaller segments).

3. Walk up one flight of stairs.

4. Eat your meals using the pacing system, pausing 30 seconds between each bite.

5. Eat at least three meals.

6. Using your Self-Monitoring tearout chart, score yourself at the end of the day for goals accomplished.

7. Review this week's progress on your chart. Are you having a difficult time accomplishing your daily goals? Is one area (decreasing fat, increasing physical activity, pacing your eating, or monitoring) more difficult than another for you? Analyze your strengths and weaknesses, and develop a strategy for overcoming any problems in your way.

8. If you have not weighed yourself yet, do so today.

DAY 8

COOKING WITHOUT FAT

Some people truly believe that a life with little fat is a life with little joy. They love the taste and the feel of fat—its moisture and its smooth texture on the tongue and the palate. But even low-fat dining can be very pleasurable. Here are some suggestions you can use to make your meals both low-fat and delectable.

- Avoid frying (which increases the food's fat content because it literally adds fat to the basic food), relying instead on methods that permit the fat to drip off during cooking—including broiling, baking, roasting, and braising. Also, remember that medium or well-done meat will tend to have less fat than rare meat, since fat continues to be lost as long as the cooking process continues. Be sure you have trimmed away all visible fat before cooking. Since lean beef cooks faster than fattier cuts, cook it for about 20 percent less time than you would cook beef that is higher in fat. Beef that is overcooked will probably be tougher than you'd like.

- Use nonstick cookware. Instead of cooking with butter, use a little nonstick cooking spray.

- Refrigerate soups, stews, and sauces before serving them. When you take them out of the refrigerator, the fat will have congealed at the top. Skim it off the surface before reheating.

- For pancake and waffle toppings, use fresh fruit (strawberries, blueberries) or applesauce. Fruit can also be added to many muffin and pancake recipes.

- Begin cooking with half the amount of fat called for in the recipe. In general, you won't need to add any more, and the chemistry of the recipe won't be significantly altered.

Vegetables with strong aromas (onions, peppers, celery, garlic) can enhance the flavor of many dishes with substantially reduced fat content.

- Use some creativity in making low-fat substitutions when preparing food. For instance, instead of putting butter on your baked potato, try salsa. Rather than cooking with whole-milk cheddar cheese, use part-skim mozzarella. For some other ideas, see "Trading Down the Fat in Your Favorite Recipes" (page 175).

DAY 8

Assignment

1. Decrease fat in your diet so it accounts for less than 20 percent of your total calories for the day. To accomplish this, increase your intake of foods that have 10 percent or less of their calories from fat and cut back significantly on foods with 30 percent or more of their calories from fat.

2. Cover 4,000 feet (walking or running at any pace, continuously or in smaller segments).

3. Walk up two flights of stairs.

4. Eat your meals using the pacing system, pausing 30 seconds between each bite.

5. Eat at least three meals.

6. Choose one of the following:

    a. Reduce the amount of fat in the next meal you cook, either by choosing a different cooking method (for example, broiling instead of frying) or by reducing the amount of fat (butter, margarine, or oil) called for in the recipe. In fact, you can reduce the fat in most recipes up to 50 percent without significantly altering the taste of the dish.

    b. Make a pasta dish today. Pasta can be a wonderfully satisfying low-fat food, as long as you avoid traditional high-fat versions of sauces such as Alfredo and pesto.

7. Using your Self-Monitoring tearout chart, score yourself at the end of the day for goals accomplished.

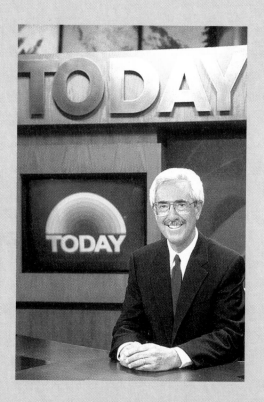

Art Ulene, M.D. (right) is the medical expert on NBC's TODAY show.

Volunteers from the Washington, D.C. area (below) participated in our weight-loss program on the TODAY show. When this photograph was taken at a reunion six months later, their average weight loss was 18.5 pounds.

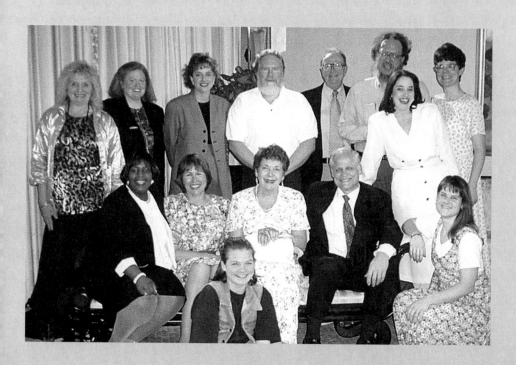

LOSE WEIGHT WITH DR. ART ULENE SELF-MONITORING CHART

Record-keeping is an important component of your success in this program. Use one of the tearout, color-coded, Self-Monitoring charts that follow to keep track of your progress. Post the chart on the refrigerator or in another conspicuous place, and at the end of each day, fill it in according to the guidelines found in Chapter 8.

Write the date of the week in the upper right-hand corner of each box. Then everyday, fill in the entire circle, half of it, or none of it, depending on how well you fared in the three areas you're monitoring. Following completion of the 28-day Plan, continue using the charts for the Continuity Phase (Chapter 11) of the program.

When filling out the circles

- Did you successfully reduce the amount of dietary fat you consumed? Use the blue circles to chart your dietary progress.

- Did you complete the exercise assignment for the day (or an equivalent physical activity)? Use the red circles.

- Did you change your eating behavior by slowing your eating pace and pausing 30 seconds between bites? Use the yellow circles.

By evaluating these charts, you'll be able to identify your patterns of success, and single out those problem areas that need special attention. The more circles you are able to fill in completely, the better!

SELF-MONITORING CHART

WEEK _____

	MONDAY	TUESDAY	WEDNESDAY	THURSDAY	FRIDAY	SATURDAY	SUNDAY
Cut Fat	○	○	○	○	○	○	○
Increase Exercise	○	○	○	○	○	○	○
Modify Behavior	○	○	○	○	○	○	○

WEEK _____

	MONDAY	TUESDAY	WEDNESDAY	THURSDAY	FRIDAY	SATURDAY	SUNDAY
Cut Fat	○	○	○	○	○	○	○
Increase Exercise	○	○	○	○	○	○	○
Modify Behavior	○	○	○	○	○	○	○

WEEK _____

	MONDAY	TUESDAY	WEDNESDAY	THURSDAY	FRIDAY	SATURDAY	SUNDAY
Cut Fat	○	○	○	○	○	○	○
Increase Exercise	○	○	○	○	○	○	○
Modify Behavior	○	○	○	○	○	○	○

WEEK _____

	MONDAY	TUESDAY	WEDNESDAY	THURSDAY	FRIDAY	SATURDAY	SUNDAY
Cut Fat	○	○	○	○	○	○	○
Increase Exercise	○	○	○	○	○	○	○
Modify Behavior	○	○	○	○	○	○	○

WEEK _____

	MONDAY	TUESDAY	WEDNESDAY	THURSDAY	FRIDAY	SATURDAY	SUNDAY
Cut Fat	○	○	○	○	○	○	○
Increase Exercise	○	○	○	○	○	○	○
Modify Behavior	○	○	○	○	○	○	○

met goal ●   partially met goal ◑   missed goal ○

SELF-MONITORING CHART

WEEK _____

	MONDAY	TUESDAY	WEDNESDAY	THURSDAY	FRIDAY	SATURDAY	SUNDAY
Cut Fat	○	○	○	○	○	○	○
Increase Exercise	○	○	○	○	○	○	○
Modify Behavior	○	○	○	○	○	○	○

WEEK _____

	MONDAY	TUESDAY	WEDNESDAY	THURSDAY	FRIDAY	SATURDAY	SUNDAY
Cut Fat	○	○	○	○	○	○	○
Increase Exercise	○	○	○	○	○	○	○
Modify Behavior	○	○	○	○	○	○	○

WEEK _____

	MONDAY	TUESDAY	WEDNESDAY	THURSDAY	FRIDAY	SATURDAY	SUNDAY
Cut Fat	○	○	○	○	○	○	○
Increase Exercise	○	○	○	○	○	○	○
Modify Behavior	○	○	○	○	○	○	○

WEEK _____

	MONDAY	TUESDAY	WEDNESDAY	THURSDAY	FRIDAY	SATURDAY	SUNDAY
Cut Fat	○	○	○	○	○	○	○
Increase Exercise	○	○	○	○	○	○	○
Modify Behavior	○	○	○	○	○	○	○

WEEK _____

	MONDAY	TUESDAY	WEDNESDAY	THURSDAY	FRIDAY	SATURDAY	SUNDAY
Cut Fat	○	○	○	○	○	○	○
Increase Exercise	○	○	○	○	○	○	○
Modify Behavior	○	○	○	○	○	○	○

met goal ●   partially met goal ◑   missed goal

SELF-MONITORING CHART

WEEK _____

	MONDAY	TUESDAY	WEDNESDAY	THURSDAY	FRIDAY	SATURDAY	SUNDAY
Cut Fat	○	○	○	○	○	○	○
Increase Exercise	○	○	○	○	○	○	○
Modify Behavior	○	○	○	○	○	○	○

WEEK _____

	MONDAY	TUESDAY	WEDNESDAY	THURSDAY	FRIDAY	SATURDAY	SUNDAY
Cut Fat	○	○	○	○	○	○	○
Increase Exercise	○	○	○	○	○	○	○
Modify Behavior	○	○	○	○	○	○	○

WEEK _____

	MONDAY	TUESDAY	WEDNESDAY	THURSDAY	FRIDAY	SATURDAY	SUNDAY
Cut Fat	○	○	○	○	○	○	○
Increase Exercise	○	○	○	○	○	○	○
Modify Behavior	○	○	○	○	○	○	○

WEEK _____

	MONDAY	TUESDAY	WEDNESDAY	THURSDAY	FRIDAY	SATURDAY	SUNDAY
Cut Fat	○	○	○	○	○	○	○
Increase Exercise	○	○	○	○	○	○	○
Modify Behavior	○	○	○	○	○	○	○

WEEK _____

	MONDAY	TUESDAY	WEDNESDAY	THURSDAY	FRIDAY	SATURDAY	SUNDAY
Cut Fat	○	○	○	○	○	○	○
Increase Exercise	○	○	○	○	○	○	○
Modify Behavior	○	○	○	○	○	○	○

met goal ●   partially met goal ◐   missed goal ○

SELF-MONITORING CHART

WEEK _____

	MONDAY	TUESDAY	WEDNESDAY	THURSDAY	FRIDAY	SATURDAY	SUNDAY
Cut Fat	○	○	○	○	○	○	○
Increase Exercise	○	○	○	○	○	○	○
Modify Behavior	○	○	○	○	○	○	○

WEEK _____

	MONDAY	TUESDAY	WEDNESDAY	THURSDAY	FRIDAY	SATURDAY	SUNDAY
Cut Fat	○	○	○	○	○	○	○
Increase Exercise	○	○	○	○	○	○	○
Modify Behavior	○	○	○	○	○	○	○

WEEK _____

	MONDAY	TUESDAY	WEDNESDAY	THURSDAY	FRIDAY	SATURDAY	SUNDAY
Cut Fat	○	○	○	○	○	○	○
Increase Exercise	○	○	○	○	○	○	○
Modify Behavior	○	○	○	○	○	○	○

WEEK _____

	MONDAY	TUESDAY	WEDNESDAY	THURSDAY	FRIDAY	SATURDAY	SUNDAY
Cut Fat	○	○	○	○	○	○	○
Increase Exercise	○	○	○	○	○	○	○
Modify Behavior	○	○	○	○	○	○	○

WEEK _____

	MONDAY	TUESDAY	WEDNESDAY	THURSDAY	FRIDAY	SATURDAY	SUNDAY
Cut Fat	○	○	○	○	○	○	○
Increase Exercise	○	○	○	○	○	○	○
Modify Behavior	○	○	○	○	○	○	○

met goal ●   partially met goal   missed goal

SELF-MONITORING CHART

WEEK _____

	MONDAY	TUESDAY	WEDNESDAY	THURSDAY	FRIDAY	SATURDAY	SUNDAY
Cut Fat	○	○	○	○	○	○	○
Increase Exercise	○	○	○	○	○	○	○
Modify Behavior	○	○	○	○	○	○	○

WEEK _____

	MONDAY	TUESDAY	WEDNESDAY	THURSDAY	FRIDAY	SATURDAY	SUNDAY
Cut Fat	○	○	○	○	○	○	○
Increase Exercise	○	○	○	○	○	○	○
Modify Behavior	○	○	○	○	○	○	○

WEEK _____

	MONDAY	TUESDAY	WEDNESDAY	THURSDAY	FRIDAY	SATURDAY	SUNDAY
Cut Fat	○	○	○	○	○	○	○
Increase Exercise	○	○	○	○	○	○	○
Modify Behavior	○	○	○	○	○	○	○

WEEK _____

	MONDAY	TUESDAY	WEDNESDAY	THURSDAY	FRIDAY	SATURDAY	SUNDAY
Cut Fat	○	○	○	○	○	○	○
Increase Exercise	○	○	○	○	○	○	○
Modify Behavior	○	○	○	○	○	○	○

WEEK _____

	MONDAY	TUESDAY	WEDNESDAY	THURSDAY	FRIDAY	SATURDAY	SUNDAY
Cut Fat	○	○	○	○	○	○	○
Increase Exercise	○	○	○	○	○	○	○
Modify Behavior	○	○	○	○	○	○	○

met goal ●   partially met goal ◑   missed goal ○

SELF-MONITORING CHART

WEEK _____

	MONDAY	TUESDAY	WEDNESDAY	THURSDAY	FRIDAY	SATURDAY	SUNDAY
Cut Fat	○	○	○	○	○	○	○
Increase Exercise	○	○	○	○	○	○	○
Modify Behavior	○	○	○	○	○	○	○

WEEK _____

	MONDAY	TUESDAY	WEDNESDAY	THURSDAY	FRIDAY	SATURDAY	SUNDAY
Cut Fat	○	○	○	○	○	○	○
Increase Exercise	○	○	○	○	○	○	○
Modify Behavior	○	○	○	○	○	○	○

WEEK _____

	MONDAY	TUESDAY	WEDNESDAY	THURSDAY	FRIDAY	SATURDAY	SUNDAY
Cut Fat	○	○	○	○	○	○	○
Increase Exercise	○	○	○	○	○	○	○
Modify Behavior	○	○	○	○	○	○	○

WEEK _____

	MONDAY	TUESDAY	WEDNESDAY	THURSDAY	FRIDAY	SATURDAY	SUNDAY
Cut Fat	○	○	○	○	○	○	○
Increase Exercise	○	○	○	○	○	○	○
Modify Behavior	○	○	○	○	○	○	○

WEEK _____

	MONDAY	TUESDAY	WEDNESDAY	THURSDAY	FRIDAY	SATURDAY	SUNDAY
Cut Fat	○	○	○	○	○	○	○
Increase Exercise	○	○	○	○	○	○	○
Modify Behavior	○	○	○	○	○	○	○

met goal 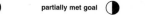 partially met goal   missed goal

DAY 9

EXERCISING
WITHOUT EXERCISING

Beyond incorporating daily walking into your life, you must also find other ways to increase your overall physical activity. Remember, the more activity you do, the more calories you will burn.

In his book *Exercise à la Carte*, Dr. George Dixon offers some excellent ideas for increasing the amount of physical activity in your life. Some of these ideas are presented here. As you look at this list, start thinking of new ways to increase your own daily activity.

- Whenever you can, forget the elevator and use the stairs instead. In high-rise buildings, get off the elevator a few floors before your stop and walk the rest of the way. (Just make sure the stairway doors allow access.)

- Park a block or two (or more) away from your job or any destination and walk the extra distance.

- When you go shopping, don't fight with other drivers for the closest spaces; instead, park at the far end of the lot, where lots of spaces are available, and walk to the store. (You'll probably get to your destination faster than you would if you spent the time circling the lot looking for the prime spot.)

- Walk whenever and wherever possible. Don't jump into the car to get milk from the neighborhood market—walk instead. Most city blocks are about a tenth of a mile long. In two trips to a market two blocks away, you'll walk eight-tenths of a mile and burn off about 80 calories.

- When you have packages to unload from your car, take them into your house one at a time to increase the number of trips back and forth.

- Invest in a cordless phone so you can talk and walk at the same time. (Think about how many feet you could cover during a half-hour call!)

- Move briskly. The faster you move, the more calories you burn during each minute you spend in the activity. Walking briskly—even if it's only for five or ten minutes—will burn more calories than taking a leisurely stroll for the same amount of time. Don't forget, though: In general it's the distance that counts; if you walk ten blocks at a slow pace, you will burn more calories than if you walk five blocks quickly.

- When you do yard work, use manual tools (hand mowers, rakes, snow shovels) instead of power tools whenever you can do it without exhausting yourself or risking injury.

- If you are at home most of the day and there are stairs in your house, take a break every hour or two and climb a flight or two of stairs. Remember: As far as weight control is concerned, it's not how many flights you walk at one time, it's how many you walk over the course of the day.

- Do more housework. Roughly half an hour of mopping the floor, sweeping, vacuuming, or general cleaning burns off 100 calories.

- Think of fun activities you can start doing every week or so. If you've always loved dancing, take a class once or twice a week. You'll be burning calories (about 200 an hour for ballroom dancing; 400 per hour for modern and square dancing). What's more, you'll reap the psychological benefits of being with other people and doing something you love. Hiking, snow skiing, waterskiing, and tennis are other excellent ways to have fun while burning excess calories.

- Renew your acquaintance with an activity you used to enjoy. Think back to when you were a kid. What were your favorite sports or activities? Did you enjoy jumping rope, participating in track events, doing gymnastics, or hiking? You can still have great fun doing these things, even though you may not be able to do them as gracefully or as well as you did in your youth.

- Create other activities around exercise. Listen to music while you walk or climb stairs.

For more information on exercise alternatives, consult *Exercise à la Carte*. (See Resources, page 317.)

DAY 9

Assignment

1. Decrease fat in your diet so it accounts for less than 20 percent of your total calories for the day. To accomplish this, increase your intake of foods that have 10 percent or less of their calories from fat and cut back significantly on foods with 30 percent or more of their calories from fat.

2. Cover 4,500 feet (walking or running at any pace, continuously or in smaller segments).

3. Walk up two flights of stairs.

4. Eat your meals using the pacing system, pausing 30 seconds between each bite.

5. Eat at least three meals.

6. Choose one of the following:

   a. When doing an errand today, walk instead of driving. (For example, walk to the cleaners or the pharmacy, or park your car in between the two and walk to both.)

   b. When watching TV today, use one-pound food cans (or barbells, if you have them), to do some strength training exercises for the upper body (see page 99).

7. Using your Self-Monitoring tearout chart, score yourself at the end of the day for goals accomplished.

DAY 10

SETTING UP YOUR SUPPORT NETWORK

For some people, trying to lose weight is a private matter. They are self-motivated and prefer to undertake their weight-loss efforts on their own. Others, however, do better with some external support.

That support can come from several sources. In a sense, this book is a source of support, providing information, inspiration, and a structured program to help you in the weeks and months ahead. But support from the people in your life can be just as important. In fact, studies show that most people trying to lose weight do better when they have a little help from their friends (and family and co-workers). Here are some ways to get that help:

- Ask your family to join your low-fat eating plan. They may agree to keep high-fat foods out of the refrigerator where they can tempt you, and they can also help out in the kitchen, preparing some of the low-fat meals you eat. When you sit down together for meals, you can help one another slow down the eating pace until pausing between bites becomes routine for all of you.

- Invite family and friends to walk with you in the morning or evening. Or ask co-workers to become your everyday exercise partners, joining you for lunchtime walks or climbing stairs with you after work.

- Rather than planning all your social gatherings around food, invite friends to join you for a tour of the museum or a visit to the park—and pack a low-fat lunch instead of going to an all-you-can-eat restaurant. Don't wait for people to offer their help. Reach out and ask for the kind of support you need. Make your requests precise. For example:

"I've found a new weight-loss program that's different than any I've seen. I think it's going to work and would love you to go through the 28 days with me. Let me give you the book to read, and then let's talk it over."

"I've 'raided' the cupboard for a late-night, high-fat snack two nights in a row. It sure would help me if you would agree to keep those snacks out of the house, or at least somewhere else in our home out of my line of sight. Can I count on you for that?"

Remind the people in your life that you're relying on their help to succeed. Be assertive. Make your requests specific but nonaccusatory: *"You can make it easier for me by not offering me a slice of the pie you bought."* Or, *"I'd like you to exercise with me, but if you'd rather not, you can help me by making the VCR available for my aerobics video workout at 7 o'clock every night."*

Keep in mind that as supportive as your family members and friends become, they are only human, and they're bound to have occasional lapses, just as you may have setbacks with this program now and then. Your usually supportive spouse may become exasperated with your slower (and healthier) eating pace and complain that you are still eating long after everyone else is done. If so, be patient, and remind him or her of the health benefits that will accompany your new behavior. When family members *are* being supportive, don't forget to thank them for improving your chances of success.

Sometimes family members and friends may *deliberately* try to sabotage your diet. There are many complex reasons for this kind of behavior. The people closest to you may become uncomfortable with the physical and psychological changes that accompany your weight loss. Your spouse may worry that if you become thinner, you'll be more attractive to the opposite sex—something he or she just can't handle. An overweight friend may fear that as a thin person, you may develop a new social network that leaves him or her behind. Family members may simply miss having an eating partner for the high-fat foods they enjoy, or they may feel jealous over your successful weight loss, particularly if they're obese themselves.

With motivations like these, the intentional sabotage can take many forms. Friends and spouses may eat high-fat foods in front of you and talk about the experience with great enthusiasm. They may invite you to share foods they know you are trying to avoid. Or they may even ridicule your weight-loss efforts and try to convince you that you really don't need to shed any weight at all.

Whether the subversion is deliberate or subconscious, you need to talk frankly with people you feel are undermining your efforts. Discuss the reasons for the sabotage: Why are they feeling insecure or anxious about your weight loss? Is there something you can do to put their fears to rest? In most cases, you can turn that sabotage into support with a frank discussion of what you see happening, and a heartfelt request for their assistance.

DAY 10

Assignment

1. Decrease fat in your diet so it accounts for less than 20 percent of your total calories for the day. To accomplish this, increase your intake of foods that have 10 percent or less of their calories from fat and cut back significantly on foods with 30 percent or more of their calories from fat.

2. Cover 5,000 feet (walking or running at any pace, continuously or in smaller segments).

3. Walk up two flights of stairs.

4. Eat your meals using the pacing system, pausing 30 seconds between each bite.

5. Eat at least three meals.

6. Choose one of the following:

   a. Invite a friend or family member to walk with you today.

   b. Discuss this weight-loss plan with your family or a friend or a co-worker, identifying ways in which they can support your efforts, and ask for their help.

7. Using your Self-Monitoring tearout chart, score yourself at the end of the day for goals accomplished.

DAY 11

EATING OUT

Many people use eating out as an excuse for not losing weight—but it is not a valid excuse. There are lots of things you can do to control the food you get in restaurants; you just have to be a little creative.

Tailor the Menu to Suit Your Needs

Just ten years ago, many restaurant waiters and chefs might have turned down special requests that required them to alter their basic recipes. Today, very few restaurants are unwilling to tailor menu items to meet your dietary needs and wishes. *But you've got to ask.*

If French fries are the standard side dish, ask for a baked potato or sliced tomato instead. Request that poultry be skinned before cooking, and have all sauces (as well as salad dressings and gravies) served on the side, so you can use them sparingly. Even if you can't find a vegetable plate on the menu, don't be afraid to ask that one be made up. A good chef at a good restaurant will make whatever effort is necessary to ensure that you're satisfied with your meal. If you don't get this kind of treatment at a restaurant, don't go back.

Skipping Starters

Try to recall the last time you ate out and ordered an appetizer. You probably didn't really need the meal that followed. Few of us require that much food to fill up. So, next time you dine out, consider skipping the appetizer completely or sharing one with a dining companion. If the appetizer menu looks more attractive than the main courses, order one appetizer to start and another as your second course. Since appetizer servings are generally smaller, you'll probably get just about the right amount of food by ordering this way.

Select Wisely

The same sensible rules you use for meals at home still apply when you are ordering meals in restaurants: Select foods that are low in fat and have them prepared in a manner that keeps them that way. Pasta is low in fat, but not when prepared with a heavy cream sauce (choose the marinara sauce instead). Chicken can be a good choice, but not when breaded and stuffed with prosciutto and cheese. Even a steak is acceptable if you order a lean cut and eat only a three- or four-ounce portion.

Here are a few examples of smart restaurant selections:

- For breakfast, order hot cereal, and ask the waiter to hold the melted butter that is usually placed on top. Many cold cereals are good choices, too, as long as you use skim milk with them (but stay away from the high-fat granolas).

- Eggs can be a good selection, but the way they are cooked and served is especially important. Order omelets with vegetables instead of cheese, and skip the side of bacon or sausage that usually accompanies the eggs.

- Pancakes and waffles are excellent choices, unless you smother them in butter or syrup. Always order the "short stack" and eat it more slowly. You'll feel just as full afterward with one-half to one-third fewer calories.

- For lunch, sandwiches can be a wise choice if you select the right fillings. Choose turkey or chicken and avoid high-fat meats like bologna, corned beef and pastrami. Skip the cheese and use mustard in place of mayonnaise whenever possible.

- Soup and salad is another good dining option if you follow certain guidelines. Stay away from the cream-based soups, use salad dressing sparingly (order it on the side), and don't put butter or margarine on the bread that is served with it. (For a delicious treat, dip the bread into the soup instead).

Choosing a Restaurant

Some kinds of cuisine are more conducive to eating "light" than others, but you can succeed at almost any type of restaurant if you try. Here are a few tips to help you enjoy different ethnic cuisines the low-fat way:

Mexican: Try a chicken tostada, but ask for the guacamole and sour cream on the side, and skip the fried tortilla in which this dish is served (okay, so it's not really a tostada any longer; but it is still delicious, much lower in calories and fat, and better for you).

Italian: Pasta is an excellent option, but choose your sauce carefully. Tomato-based sauces are generally a good choice, but check to be sure the sauce is not loaded with oil. A good Italian chef can make a tasty tomato sauce without any oil (but many will not do so unless you ask for it this way). And remember to go light on the Parmesan cheese.

French: French restaurants—notorious for their high-fat sauces—need not be avoided, but you will have to be selective in choosing dishes, and you should ask if the sauces can be served on the side. Roasted chicken can be found on most French menus and is a wise choice, provided you request that the skin be removed (preferably before it is cooked). Also, ask for a serving of fresh or cooked vegetables instead of the pomme frites (French fries) that are traditionally served.

Japanese: Japanese restaurants typically feature many low-fat menu options. Select steamed or stir-fried chicken or fish, and plain rice instead of deep-fried dishes such as tempura. Sushi can also be a good choice if you're careful to avoid fatty fish such as eel and mackerel.

Chinese: Choose a vegetarian entree or one containing skinless chicken or fish instead of beef. Be aware, however, that many of the sauces in Chinese restaurants are quite high in fat. Select your sauce carefully or order stir-fried dishes without sauces. Eat lots of steamed rice and go easy on the dishes containing meats.

Remove the Temptation

How many times have you eaten more than you wanted to only because the food was there in front of you? This can be a particular problem when dining out, because it's usually the waiter who decides when the plates will be cleared—which means you could be staring at some very tempting food long after you've had enough to eat. You can change that. As soon as you've eaten as much as you want, ask the waiter to take your plate. And don't feel compelled to clean your plate just because you're paying for it. If you've left a significant amount of food, ask for a doggy bag and enjoy a "free" meal at home the next day.

Another great way to remove temptation is to leave it in the kitchen, especially in restaurants that are known for large portions. Simply ask the waiter—at the time you're placing your order—to serve only half of your meal, and to put the other half in a take-home container. Keep that container in the kitchen until you are ready to leave; you won't eat what you can't see.

The same rules apply to things like bread and butter. My rule is: If the bread in a restaurant isn't good enough to be eaten without butter, it shouldn't be eaten at all. So, ask the waiter to remove the butter or margarine from the table. If you insist on using butter or margarine, put a small amount of spread on your bread plate, and then have the rest taken away from the table.

Dealing with Dessert

Even after you've safely navigated your way through a low-fat meal, the waiter may present you with a list of mouth-watering desserts. For those of us with a sweet tooth, this is when the really tough decisions are made. If you're full from dinner, the best thing you can do at this point is say, "No, thank you." It may be difficult getting the words out on the first few occasions (and you may even sense that something is "missing" from your meal), but each time you eat out it will get a little easier. Ultimately, skipping dessert will feel natural and painless.

If, on the other hand, you've left room for dessert or you've "banked" some calories ahead of time (see page 222), here are some tips to help you order wisely:

- Order a gourmet coffee, like cappuccino, as your dessert (be sure to have it made with nonfat milk and skip the whipped cream). This will help fill the "void" at the end of the meal and, if you top it with a little ground chocolate, satisfy your sweet tooth.

- Order one dessert, but request extra forks or spoons for everyone at the table. This will provide you with the "dessert experience" at only a fraction of the calories.

- Order fresh fruit or sorbet.

DAY 11

Assignment

1. Decrease fat in your diet so it accounts for less than 20 percent of your total calories for the day. To accomplish this, increase your intake of foods that have 10 percent or less of their calories from fat and cut back significantly on foods with 30 percent or more of their calories from fat.

2. Cover 5,500 feet (walking or running at any pace, continuously or in smaller segments).

3. Walk up two flights of stairs.

4. Eat your meals using the pacing system, pausing 30 seconds between each bite.

5. Eat at least three meals.

6. Choose one of the following:

   a. Go out to eat and order a delicious low-fat meal, like grilled fish or pasta with fresh tomato and garlic. Don't hesitate to request "no fat" in the cooking. Most chefs are happy to do this.

   b. Reward yourself today if you've been following the program. After eating out, take yourself to the movies or buy that book you've been wanting.

7. Using your Self-Monitoring tearout chart, score yourself at the end of the day for goals accomplished.

DAY 12

TRADING DOWN THE FAT IN YOUR FAVORITE RECIPES

Even though you're decreasing the amount of fat you eat, you don't need to throw out higher-fat recipes that might have been family favorites for years.

Three strategies can help you "have your cake and eat it, too":

- **Dilution**: thinning out the high-fat foods you eat by, for example, cooking with extenders

- **Diminution**: decreasing portion size

- **Substitution**: replacing high-fat foods with low-fat alternatives

Food extenders, for example, are low-fat ingredients that can be mixed into your favorite dishes, and thus they can "stretch" a primary ingredient that may be high in fat. So while you can still enjoy the primary ingredient, each serving will contain less fat (as long as you keep the serving size the same).

Good food extenders include vegetables, fruits, beans, lentils, and grains. Many people add them to meat dishes, thus reducing the amount of meat (and fat) per serving. Incorporating carrots, potatoes, and tomatoes into a meat recipe, for instance, will cut down your fat intake, but won't sacrifice the robust nature of the dish that you might enjoy. With a meat-based soup, add beans and lentils to dramatically decrease the amount of meat you use.

You can modify your favorite recipes using the following chart of exchanges as a guide, which will help you move away from high-fat ingredients toward low-fat alternatives. Also included are some snack and side dish substitutions. In most cases, decreasing your fat intake won't mean sacrificing taste or pleasure, particularly once your palate has become accustomed to low-fat dining.

EXCHANGES

In place of these ingredients:	*Try these:*
Whole milk	Skim milk
Whole-milk cheese	Part-skim, fat-free cheese
Regular ground beef	Extra-lean ground beef
Roast beef	Roast chicken
Pork spare ribs	Lean pork loin (trimmed, broiled)
Beef hot dog	Turkey hot dog
Butter, margarine	Diet or reduced fat spreads, jam, jelly
Sour cream	Plain nonfat yogurt
Ice cream	Frozen nonfat yogurt
Doughnut, croissant	Bagel
Bologna sandwich	Sliced turkey sandwich
Buttered oil-popped popcorn	Unbuttered air-popped popcorn
Chocolate chip cookies	Fig bars
Potato chips	Pretzels
Mayonnaise	Nonfat mayonnaise, mustard

DAY 12

Assignment

1. Decrease fat in your diet so it accounts for less than 20 percent of your total calories for the day. To accomplish this, increase your intake of foods that have 10 percent or less of their calories from fat and cut back significantly on foods with 30 percent or more of their calories from fat.

2. Cover 6,000 feet (walking or running at any pace, continuously or in smaller segments).

3. Walk up two flights of stairs.

4. Eat your meals using the pacing system, pausing 30 seconds between each bite.

5. Eat at least three meals.

6. Choose one of the following:

   a. If you're an egg eater, try a low-fat omelet today. Discard the egg yolks and use only the whites. Add nonfat milk, chopped vegetables, herbs, and spices. Cook the omelet without butter or margarine in a nonstick pan, or use nonstick cooking spray.

   b. Try a microwave baked potato for lunch or dinner today. Prepare it the low-fat way: Fill it with chives, other favorite vegetables, herbs, spices, salsa, or nonfat yogurt.

7. Using your Self-Monitoring tearout chart, score yourself at the end of the day for goals accomplished.

DAY 13

FINDING TIME TO EXERCISE

For years, you've probably heard that to make your exercise sessions worthwhile, you need to engage in at least 20 to 30 minutes of continuous (aerobic) activity. While that recommendation is true if your goal is cardiovascular fitness, the guidelines are quite different when trying to lose weight. In fact, the daily exercise assignments in this book do not have to be completed at one time, but can be spread out over the course of a day. Today's assignment, for example, which is to cover 6,500 feet by walking or running, can be accomplished all at once, or in two 3,250-feet workout periods, or in four 1,625-feet segments, or even in 20 segments of 325 feet each. As long as you ultimately cover the whole 6,500 feet, you'll burn essentially the same number of calories—no matter how you divide it up or how long it takes.

This approach will make it much easier to fit exercise into your life. People often complain to me that they don't have enough time for exercise in their busy schedules. That's the same excuse I used to give, but—in my case, at least—it was a phony excuse. The real truth was that I hadn't made exercise a priority. We all can find time for things that are important to us. And when you are prepared to say that exercise is an important priority, you will find time to do it—just like I did.

One trick that will make this easier is to keep an appointment book or calendar, and block time for your exercise sessions in the same way you would make time for an appointment with your doctor or dentist. Write in all of your exercise sessions first, then build the rest of your schedule around them.

The surprising thing you will discover about exercise is that it actually creates *more* time in your day. You feel better and have more energy, so you become more effective in your work and you get more things done. Since I started exercising, I get up earlier,

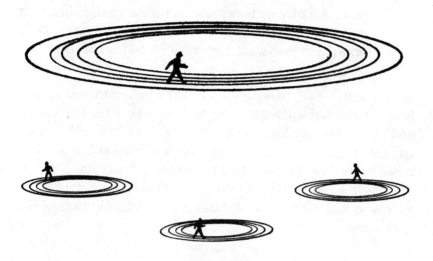

Your daily exercise assignment does not need to be done all at one time. Whether you cover the recommended walking distance in multiple mini-sessions (represented by the small ovals) or in one long session (the large oval), you'll achieve the same benefits.

stay up later, and feel more energetic throughout the day. I also sleep better on the days that I exercise.

So, if your problem (or excuse) is lack of time, here are some ideas that will help you find the time you need to increase the physical activity in your life:

- Spread your exercise out into several increments during the day instead of one long chunk of time; this way, you'll be able to more easily fit the activity into your schedule.

- Walking 500 feet takes only about two minutes. So take two minutes—or four, or six—during your coffee breaks, after lunch, or before dinner to walk 500 feet, or 1,000 or 1,500.

- Get up ten minutes earlier and stay awake ten minutes later. Believe me, spending those 20 minutes out of bed will become easier as you start exercising. Just ten minutes on both ends will create enough time for a meaningful exercise program that can help you maintain control over your weight regulator—and your weight.

- If you find it easier to do your daily assignments all at one time, you may do better setting aside a specific time each day for exercise, such as first thing in the morning. Find a time that is predictable, controllable, and not likely to conflict with other activities.

Look at it this way: Walking 1,000 feet at a brisk pace takes about four minutes and will burn about 20 calories. Do it ten times a day and you've burned 200 extra calories. Walk 1,000 feet 15 times a day (or, if you prefer, take a larger block of time and walk three miles in one stretch), and you'll be burning off an extra 300 calories daily. If you continue walking like this over the course of a year, you will burn off a total of 109,500 extra calories, which equals about 31 pounds.

DAY 13

Assignment

1. Decrease fat in your diet so it accounts for less than 20 percent of your total calories for the day. To accomplish this, increase your intake of foods that have 10 percent or less of their calories from fat and cut back significantly on foods with 30 percent or more of their calories from fat.

2. Cover 6,500 feet (walking or running at any pace, continuously or in smaller segments).

3. Walk up two flights of stairs.

4. Eat your meals using the pacing system, pausing 30 seconds between each bite.

5. Eat at least three meals.

6. Choose one of the following:

   a. If you keep a daily calendar or datebook, write an appointment for exercise into the next 30 days. Every seven days, take a moment to add another week's worth of exercise appointments to your calendar or datebook. Treat these appointments as if they were just as important as any others on your schedule. They are.

   b. Try a different time of day for all or part of your walk.

7. Using your Self-Monitoring tearout chart, score yourself at the end of the day for goals accomplished.

DAY 14

MEASURING SELF-WORTH ON THE SCALE

For some people who are trying to lose weight, the bathroom scale is a friend. It provides objective evidence of weight loss—or lack of it. The scale lets them know which weight-loss techniques are working and which are not. It motivates them to continue their program.

For others, the scale is their worst enemy. These people use the scale to measure not only their weight, but their self-worth. They lose a pound or two, and they feel good about themselves. They gain a pound or two, and they feel worthless. Their trips to the bathroom scale are an emotional roller coaster.

Separating Your Weight From Your Self-Worth

If you allow your weight to define your value as a human being, you will ride that roller coaster, too. Each day, as your weight goes up and down in its normal rhythm, your self-esteem will go up and down with it.

You are not your weight on the scale, and you must not let that weight define your worth. You are a valuable human being whose value has nothing to do with your weight or the measurement of your waist. If you find it impossible to separate your feelings of self-worth from the reading on your scale, you should just stop weighing yourself. It's only when you accept your own value that you can put this (or any other) weight-loss program into proper perspective, and begin to lose pounds that you can keep off.

Believing In and Caring About Yourself

Research shows that your beliefs and attitudes about yourself and about your ability to lose weight can have a significant influence

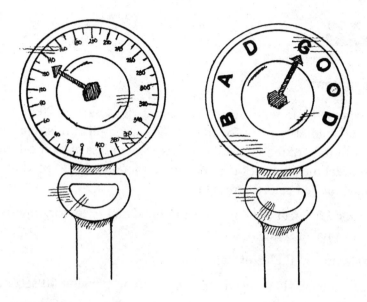

The scale is a measure only of your weight (as the first illustration shows). But, too often, people translate the number on the scale into how they feel about themselves (as in the second drawing). Don't let the scale become a reflection of your self-worth.

on whether you succeed at losing weight and keeping it off. Unfortunately, many people who are trying to lose weight have strong negative feelings about themselves. In part, these feelings grow out of the stigma our culture attaches to being overweight. (There *was* a time when obesity was considered attractive and desirable.) These feelings also develop from the frustration, guilt, and sense of failure that repeated dieting can produce.

It is time now to put any negative feelings from these past experiences behind you. You are starting a new program and a new path, and you are now finished with dieting. It is not possible to fail on your new program, because no one is keeping score. A gain in weight is not a value judgment about you; it is simply a consequence of the activities you have chosen to do.

I wish you success in your weight-loss efforts. But I want to remind you that you are already a success. Whatever the outcome of your efforts with this program, nothing can take away your value as a person—ever.

DAY 14

Assignment

1. Decrease fat in your diet so it accounts for less than 20 percent of your total calories for the day. To accomplish this, increase your intake of foods that have 10 percent or less of their calories from fat and cut back significantly on foods with 30 percent or more of their calories from fat.

2. Cover 7,000 feet (walking or running at any pace, continuously or in smaller segments).

3. Walk up two flights of stairs.

4. Eat your meals using the pacing system, pausing 30 seconds between each bite.

5. Eat at least three meals.

6. Using your Self-Monitoring tearout chart, score yourself at the end of the day for goals accomplished.

7. Review this week's progress on your chart. Are you having a difficult time accomplishing your daily goals? Is one area (decreasing fat, increasing physical activity, pacing your eating, or monitoring) more difficult than another for you? Analyze your strengths and weaknesses and develop a strategy for overcoming any problems in your way.

8. Weigh yourself today.

DAY 15

BAKING WITHOUT FAT

Believe it or not, you don't have to stop baking to lose weight. However, you may need to change the way you bake. Most baked goods derive more than 30 percent of their calories from fat (many are closer to 50 percent!). One popular brand of chocolate chip cookies, for instance, gets 46 percent of its calories from fat; a popular name-brand pound cake is 50 percent fat. To lose weight and still enjoy fresh baked goods, you have to cut this number in half—even farther, whenever possible.

Many people say they would rather give up baked goods entirely than try a low-fat variety. But, read on and you'll learn ways to reduce the fat in your favorite baking recipes without compromising on taste.

The simplest way to reduce the amount of fat when baking is to substitute reduced-fat products for high-fat ones. For example, a cheesecake that calls for four eight-ounce blocks of cream cheese can be made with four eight-ounce blocks of *fat-free* cream cheese. That single change reduces the number of calories in the finished product by 2,400—almost all of them from fat. Reduced fat margarine and "light" butter can be used in recipes instead of regular margarine and real butter. This saves you between 40 and 95 calories per tablespoon (depending on which brand you select). In a recipe that calls for a cup of heavy cream, use a cup of half-and-half and save yourself over 500 calories (use non-fat milk and the calorie count falls 230 calories more).

Another simple way to eliminate the fat from baked goods: Use naturally low-fat ingredients to replace the fats you're eliminating from the recipe. Following are a few of the natural substitutes for fat that registered dietitian Sandra Woodruff recommends in her book, *Secrets of Fat-Free Baking*, published by Avery Publishing Group, Inc. (see Resources, page 317).

Fruit substitutes. Fruit purées like applesauce and mashed bananas and fruit juices such as orange, apple, and pineapple can be used instead of fats like butter, margarine, and oil. They not only lend flavor and sweetness to baked recipes, but add important vitamins and minerals as well. (Peach purée, for example, contains large amounts of beta carotene; orange juice is rich in vitamin C; and banana purée has lots of potassium.)

Dairy substitutes. Dairy products like low-fat and nonfat yogurt, buttermilk and nonfat milk also make excellent substitutions for fats. In addition to reducing the fat, they add important nutrients like calcium and vitamin D.

Liquid sweeteners. Liquid sweeteners like honey and molasses can be successfully used in place of butter, margarine, and oil in many recipes. Although most liquid sweeteners are high in calories, they are less caloric than the fats they replace, and they also allow you to cut down on the amount of other sweeteners in the recipe.

Select a fat substitute that is compatible with your recipe. Look at the ingredients in your recipe and consider what flavors would blend in best. For example, applesauce might work nicely in bran muffins; molasses in spice cakes; and yogurt in puddings. Start by replacing only half the fat in your recipe. If you like the results, keep reducing the fat a little more each time you bake the recipe until you find the lowest level of fat you can attain without diminishing the taste or "feel" of the dish.

Guidelines for Fat Substitutions

Fruit purées and fruit juices. Replace all or part of the butter or margarine with half as much fruit juice or fruit purée. For example, if a recipe calls for 1 cup of butter, substitute all of the butter for 1/2 cup of fat substitute or replace half of the butter with 1/4 cup of fat substitute.

If the recipe calls for oil, replace all or part of the oil with 3/4 as much fat substitute. In a recipe that calls for 1 cup of oil, for instance, replace all of the oil with 3/4 cup of fat substitute, or

COMMON HIGH-FAT INGREDIENTS
USED IN BAKED GOODS

		Total Calories	Fat Calories
Oil	1 cup	1,900	1,900
Butter	1 cup	800	800
Margarine	1 cup	800	800
Shortening	1 cup	1,812	1,812

GOOD SUBSTITUTES
FOR HIGH-FAT INGREDIENTS

		Total Calories	Fat Calories
Applesauce	1 cup	100	5
Apple juice	1 cup	120	0
Orange juice	1 cup	112	5
Nonfat yogurt	1 cup	160	0
Buttermilk	1 cup	100	20
Nonfat milk	1 cup	86	4
Honey	1 cup	1,031	0
Molasses	1 cup	875	0
Maple syrup	1 cup	825	8

replace one half of the oil with about ⅜ cup of fat substitute. If the batter seems too dry, add more fat substitute.

- *Replace one cup of oil (1,900 calories, 100 percent from fat) with ¾ cup of unsweetened applesauce (75 calories, 5 percent from fat) and save 1,825 calories.*

Non-fat yogurt, buttermilk, and non-fat milk. Replace all or part of the butter or margarine with half as much dairy fat substitute. If the recipe calls for oil, replace all or part of the oil with three-fourths as much dairy fat substitute.

- *Substitute ¾ cup of buttermilk (75 calories, 20 percent from fat) for 1 cup of oil and save 1,825 calories.*

Liquid sweeteners. Replace all or part of the butter or margarine in the recipe with half as much liquid sweetener. If the recipe calls for oil, replace all or part of the oil with an equal amount of liquid sweetener. To prevent oversweetening, decrease the amount of sugar you use by the amount of liquid sweetener added. (For example, in a recipe that calls for 2 cups of sugar, if you've replaced 1 cup of oil with 1 cup of honey, use only 1 cup of sugar.)

- *Use 1 cup of molasses (875 calories, 0 percent from fat) instead of 1 cup of oil and save 1,025 calories. Since this allows you to reduce the amount of sugar you use by 1 cup, you save an additional 775 calories.*

DAY 15

Assignment

1. Decrease fat in your diet so it accounts for less than 20 percent of your total calories for the day. To accomplish this, increase your intake of foods that have 10 percent or less of their calories from fat and cut back significantly on foods with 30 percent or more of their calories from fat.

2. Cover 7,500 feet (walking or running at any pace, continuously or in smaller segments).

3. Walk up three flights of stairs.

4. Eat your meals using the pacing system, pausing 30 seconds between each bite.

5. Eat at least three meals.

6. Choose one of the following:

   a. Using the preceeding tips, create a low-fat version of one of your favorite dessert recipes.

   b. If you don't feel like baking today, treat yourself—go out for a low-fat dessert such as frozen yogurt or sorbet.

7. Using your Self-Monitoring tearout chart, score yourself at the end of the day for goals accomplished.

DAY 16

EXERCISE EXCUSES

Even if you love to exercise, there will be days when watching television or reading a good book sounds more appealing than taking your daily walk. On days like this, you'll probably be able to come up with a legitimate-sounding reason for why you shouldn't exercise. I've come up with at least a thousand excuses myself. But, keep in mind, they are just that—excuses. Other than illness and injury, there are very few valid reasons not to stick to your workout routine.

Top Exercise Excuses

Here's a list of some of the most popular excuses for not exercising, along with some ways to overcome them:

I didn't get enough sleep, and I'm too tired to exercise. Exercise is the best thing you can do for your energy level when you're tired. Exercising will revitalize you, whereas sitting around will only compound your fatigue.

Some people try to avoid exercising when they haven't gotten enough sleep, because they find exercise more difficult to do when they're tired. The fact is, after a poor night's sleep your legs may feel heavier and more sluggish than usual. But this is not the time to skip your workout. Just expect a little less from yourself and adjust your workout accordingly. If you usually jog, walk briskly. If you typically cover three miles, go only two. Setting limited goals on these days will make it easier to get started, and a partial workout is always preferable to no workout at all.

I'm expecting a phone call, so I can't leave the house. There's almost always a reason you need to be home—whether it's a phone call you're expecting, a delivery you're waiting for, or a repair person who's working in the house. If you must receive a call, schedule it before or after your workout. And make appointments for home repairs at times that won't interfere with your exercise plans. If you're expecting a package, leave a note authorizing the delivery person to leave the parcel at the door so you don't have to wait at home for it.

It upsets my stomach to exercise after I eat. If exercising after eating makes you uncomfortable, set up your schedule so your workouts always precede your meals (consider making exercise the very first thing you do after you wake up). If you happen to be hungry when it's time to exercise, try a light snack like half an apple or a piece of toast to tide you over until after your workout.

I've got appointments from early in the morning until late at night. Many people are so busy with work, they have little time to do anything else—let alone exercise. You'll always find time to exercise, however—if it's important enough to you.

The best way to get around this problem is to schedule exercise as your first appointment every day. Start scheduling the rest of your day only after you've set aside time to exercise. Don't make the mistake of trying to squeeze exercise into the empty blocks of time

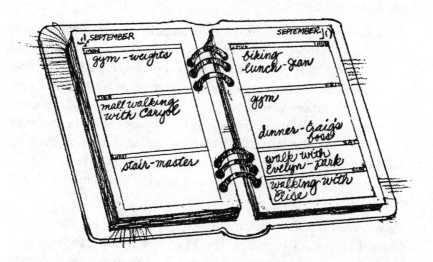

Schedule your exercise sessions just as you would other appointments. Write them in your appointment book before other commitments fill up your day.

that remain in your schedule. Those empty blocks have a way of disappearing, leaving you disappointed and out of shape.

I had to travel to another city, and it's not safe to exercise where the hotel is located. Travel can present many excuses for not exercising—from the safety of the neighborhood surrounding your hotel to the fact that you "forgot" your workout clothes at home. But travel excuses can all be avoided with a little planning. One of the most helpful strategies is to stay at a hotel that offers access to workout facilities. Most larger hotels now have fitness facilities on-site; others have agreements with nearby gyms. This solves your safety concerns and eliminates the "weather" excuse (you're guaranteed good weather indoors).

It's raining, so I can't run. Ordinarily, we go to great effort to keep ourselves dry, usually for good reasons (we're dressed for work, for example). But there's no need to stay dry when you exercise (you head straight for the shower, anyhow, after you exercise). So, if it's just drizzling (and a big storm isn't looming), you should consider exercising outdoors anyway. You'll stay warm and relatively dry if you wear a vinyl or gortex outer layer and one or more soft inner layers. Wear a baseball cap or visor to keep the rain out of your eyes.

If it's raining heavily or if it's cold outside, it's probably a good idea to stay indoors. (If you get very wet while exercising in cold weather your body temperature can drop dangerously low.) Prepare ahead for rainy days with indoor exercise alternatives. Among the choices you should consider are: using a video exercise program; walking in an enclosed shopping mall; purchasing a one-day lesson at a local fitness facility; going out for an evening of dancing—or staying in and dancing to your favorite music. By the way, all of these are good choices when it's extremely hot outside, too.

It's too cold out. You're unlikely to get too cold exercising outdoors if you dress properly. The key steps to take: Protect your hands with gloves or mittens; wear a hat to prevent loss of body heat from your head; and layer your clothes (you can remove an outer layer if you get too hot).

Cold weather can actually present some interesting exercise opportunities—cross-country skiing and snow shoeing, for example. Just walking through the snow can be fun (and excellent exercise) provided you have the proper footwear. If you live in a particularly cold environment, consider purchasing a seasonal gym membership. This will provide you with a warm workout haven on the coldest days of winter (or those days you just can't face the outdoors) and a good way to vary your exercise routine.

It's too hot out. Hot weather can be just as bad for your exercise routine as cold weather, if not worse. The thought of expending more energy than you absolutely have to on a hot day is never an appealing one. But there are a number of things you can do to maintain (and enjoy) your exercise routine through the summer.

Schedule your workouts very early in the morning or in the evening (before it gets dark) to avoid the hottest times of the day. Wear clothing that is lightweight and loose-fitting. Your best fabric choices are those that breathe, including cotton, nylon, and polypropylene. Avoid all rubberized clothing; it traps moisture and heat, and can cause your body temperature to rise dangerously. Use hot weather as an excuse to try out new types of exercise like swimming and water aerobics. Also, look for indoor exercise opportunities in buildings that are air-conditioned.

My weight regulator tricked me into skipping exercise today. A weight regulator that's malfunctioning will try to prevent you from exercising every day. It will help you dream up terrific excuses for not exercising, but if you let these excuses keep you from doing physical activity, your exercise program will never get started. So it is essential to override these initial urges to resist exercising. If you're having trouble, remind yourself how good you will feel after the exercise is over.

On the other hand, once you do get a regular activity program under way, there are going to be days when you really don't feel like exercising. These are actually important days to take off from your exercise routine. By forcing yourself to exercise when you really don't want to, you will condition yourself to dread exercising altogether.

However, when you decide to take off a day, don't let it turn into two or three. The longer you go without exercising, the harder it will be to get back into your daily routine. On days when you don't exercise, look for ways to increase the amount of other physical activity you do. Make it fun though, so it doesn't feel like exercise. Spend a few minutes gardening, for example, or go to the park and fly a kite.

DAY 16

Assignment

1. Decrease fat in your diet so it accounts for less than 20 percent of your total calories for the day. To accomplish this, increase your intake of foods that have 10 percent or less of their calories from fat and cut back significantly on foods with 30 percent or more of their calories from fat.

2. Cover 8,000 feet (walking or running at any pace, continuously or in smaller segments).

3. Walk up three flights of stairs.

4. Eat your meals using the pacing system, pausing 30 seconds between each bite.

5. Eat at least three meals.

6. Choose one of the following:

   a. Make walking a social activity. Invite a friend or a coworker to join you. A walk is a perfect opportunity for conversation; take advantage of it.

   b. Vary your walking route today. Try a different path in your own neighborhood, or drive to a scenic location and take your walk there. Variety increases your enjoyment and helps you to maintain interest in exercising.

7. Using your Self-Monitoring tearout chart, score yourself at the end of the day for goals accomplished.

DAY 17

TEN KEYS TO MODIFYING YOUR EATING BEHAVIORS

In addition to the changes you're making in dietary choices and exercise habits, behavior modification strategies can assist in your weight-loss success. Here are the key behavior changes that can help you in the days and weeks ahead:

1. In the supermarket, use a detailed shopping list and shop on a full stomach; this will help avoid impulse purchases.

2. Eat all of your meals at one place in your home. Choose a site such as the dining room, away from the kitchen.

3. Use smaller plates on your dining table. They will make food portions seem larger than they are. Keep serving bowls off the table, where they might tempt you to reach for another helping in mid-meal.

4. When dining, keep your attention focused only on eating. Avoid reading or watching TV, and enjoy the taste, texture and other sensations of the food. You'll eat less when this happens.

5. Consume your food slowly. As well as slowing the pace of your chewing, place your fork down between bites and wait 30 seconds before picking up the fork again and taking the next bite.

6. If you want a second helping, wait five minutes before deciding whether to get up and place it on your plate.

7. Leave the table as soon as you have finished eating. Immediately put leftovers in opaque containers and store them out of your line of sight.

8. Ask family and friends to support you in your weight-loss efforts. They can provide the encouragement you need to succeed.

9. Examine your chart at least once a week, using it to pinpoint problems that could be interfering with your progress.

10. Provide yourself with rewards for following the program. By making these rewards personally meaningful, they will help you stick with the plan.

DAY 17

Assignment

1. Decrease fat in your diet so it accounts for less than 20 percent of your total calories for the day. To accomplish this, increase your intake of foods that have 10 percent or less of their calories from fat and cut back significantly on foods with 30 percent or more of their calories from fat.

2. Cover 8,500 feet (walking or running at any pace, continuously or in smaller segments).

3. Walk up three flights of stairs.

4. Eat your meals using the pacing system, pausing 30 seconds between each bite.

5. Eat at least three meals.

6. Choose one of the following:

   a. Try a new low-fat or nonfat food today in place of a high-fat product that you used to eat. It's important to vary your diet to keep it interesting.

   b. Reward yourself today for following the program: Buy yourself a new piece of clothing or a bouquet of fresh flowers.

7. Using your Self-Monitoring tearout chart, score yourself at the end of the day for goals accomplished.

DAY 18

LOW-FAT PARTIES, CELEBRATIONS & HOLIDAYS

If you're not careful, the food served at social events can rapidly undermine your weight-loss plan. Trays of hors d'oeuvres, multiple course meals, and rich desserts can derail your otherwise conscientious efforts at low-fat eating.

But it doesn't have to be that way. Plan ahead, eat and drink with your weight-loss goals in mind, and you can stay on track without feeling you've missed out on having a good time at the party.

Here are some tips that will help you stay on course when you're invited to a social gathering:

- Eat lightly and wisely before you leave for the party so you don't arrive with an empty stomach. You'll find it much easier to eat lightly and thoughtfully throughout the event.

- Bring a low-fat dish of your own to the party to share with everyone else. If your dish is the only good choice for you at the buffet, don't hesitate to fill up your own plate with it. Leave a little room for tasting small portions of other dishes, so you don't feel deprived of anything.

- When you are not specifically going to get food, keep your distance from the table where the food is being served. If you stand next to it all night long, you'll almost inevitably eat more.

- Avoid the sauces, the gravies, and the high-fat dips. Ask that your salad dressing and other toppings be served on the side.

- Don't overeat just to please your host. Be stingy with your portions and generous with your compliments.

- Eat slowly, and don't feel as though you have to finish everything on your plate.

- Limit your alcohol intake. Decide in advance how much you're going to drink; once you've reached your quota, switch to non-alcoholic beverages such as diet sodas or water. Alcohol contains lots of calories, and it can impair your ability to stay in control of what you eat.

- When giving a party, be sure to offer your guests (and yourself) plenty of low-fat food options and non-alcoholic beverage choices. You'll be surprised how many of your guests will choose these over the traditional high-fat, high-calorie fare. If you're concerned about the taste and appearance of the dishes you'll be serving, visit your local bookstore. You'll find dozens of cookbooks that are filled with delicious low-fat recipes for visually appealing party food.

DAY 18

Assignment

1. Decrease fat in your diet so it accounts for less than 20 percent of your total calories for the day. To accomplish this, increase your intake of foods that have 10 percent or less of their calories from fat and cut back significantly on foods with 30 percent or more of their calories from fat.

2. Cover 9,000 feet (walking or running at any pace, continuously or in smaller segments).

3. Walk up three flights of stairs.

4. Eat your meals using the pacing system, pausing 30 seconds between each bite.

5. Eat at least three meals.

6. Choose one of the following:

   a. Invite some friends over for dinner tonight. Plan a complete low-fat meal (don't say a word, and they'll never know the difference).

   b. Go to a bookstore and buy a low-fat cookbook that includes foods for entertaining.

7. Using your Self-Monitoring tearout chart, score yourself at the end of the day for goals accomplished.

DAY 19

THE STORY ON CARBOHYDRATES

I've already described how cutting back on fat can help you regain control of your weight regulator. But one other point deserves particular attention: As you seek replacements for the high-fat foods you've been eating, your best choices are carbohydrates—especially complex carbohydrates.

Many foods fall into the carbohydrate category. The most simple carbohydrates are sugars such as fructose (the sugar in most fruits) and sucrose (table sugar). While these carbohydrates do provide necessary energy for your body, they don't have much (if any) additional nutritional value. On the other hand, complex carbohydrates—like beans, pasta, and potatoes—are rich sources of nutrients. Spaghetti, for example, supplies protein, iron, niacin, riboflavin, phosphorus, and magnesium, and dried beans are a good source of iron, potassium, and protein.

There is yet another reason to concentrate on carbohydrates and get away from fat: Carbohydrates are more satisfying than fat. Studies show that people fed carbohydrate-rich meals eat less and consume fewer calories than those fed high-fat meals. Eating carbohydrates at the beginning of a meal appears to be particularly helpful, causing you to fill up and stop eating sooner.

Can't Carbohydrates Make You Fat, Too?

Any type of food can make you fat if you eat too much of it, and carbohydrates are no exception. Although carbohydrates are a better choice than fat, you can overdo your intake of carbohydrates. Here's why: Your body prefers to burn carbohydrates for fuel before it starts to burn fat (which is what you must burn to lose weight that stays off for the long term). For instance, if you consume 1,500 calories of carbohydrates in a day, your body will

FIBER

Fiber is a special type of complex carbohydrate that is found only in plant food. Although fiber provides the body with no nutrients in its own right (it is actually indigestible as it passes through the intestine), it offers enormous health benefits. High levels of fiber intake have been associated with a decreased risk of heart disease, colon cancer, diabetes, and constipation. Fiber is also helpful when you are trying to lose weight. Not only are fiber-rich foods generally low in fat, but they are filling and they tend to require more chewing, so they make you eat more slowly. High-fiber foods also reduce blood levels of insulin, a hormone that can stimulate the appetite.

Most Americans do not consume nearly as much fiber as they should. Although government guidelines recommend a daily intake of 20 to 30 grams of fiber per day, the diets of most American men and women include only about 12 grams a day. These low levels of fiber intake may help explain why so many people are overweight.

---

burn those carbohydrates first before it begins to burn the fat you've eaten. If only 1,500 calories are required to meet your energy needs for the day, they will all come from the carbohydrates you have eaten, so all of the fat you consume that day will be stored in your body as fat.

If you consume 2,000 calories of carbohydrates, and your body needs only 1,500 calories of fuel that day, you'll have an excess of 500 calories of carbohydrates (in addition to the fat calories you consume). What happens to those 500 extra carbohydrate calories? Your body tries to store them, but first it turns some of that carbohydrate into fat. This process is not a one-to-one conversion—that is, your body will not turn the 500 calories of excess carbohydrates into 500 calories of stored fat. But it may convert a portion of those extra carbohydrates into, perhaps, 50 calories of stored fat. So, you should move in the direction of replacing the fat in your diet with carbohydrates, but don't consume those carbohydrates in an unlimited way.

DAY 19

Assignment

1. Decrease fat in your diet so it accounts for less than 20 percent of your total calories for the day. To accomplish this, increase your intake of foods that have 10 percent or less of their calories from fat and cut back significantly on foods with 30 percent or more of their calories from fat.

2. Cover 9,500 feet (walking or running at any pace, continuously or in smaller segments).

3. Walk up three flights of stairs.

4. Eat your meals using the pacing system, pausing 30 seconds between each bite.

5. Eat at least three meals.

6. Choose one of the following:

   a. Include complex carbohydrates such as potatoes, pasta, or beans in at least two of your meals today.

   b. In addition to your walking assignment, increase your activity level today by doing something fun: Make a tennis date, go for a swim, go horseback riding, go out dancing.

7. Using your Self-Monitoring tearout chart, score yourself at the end of the day for goals accomplished.

DAY 20

ALCOHOL

For someone trying to lose weight, alcohol can cause problems in several ways. Alcohol is highly caloric. A 12-ounce bottle of beer contains about 150 calories, a four-ounce glass of wine has about 90 calories, and two ounces of whiskey, gin, or vodka deliver about 140 calories. This may not sound like much, but consider what happens if you have one drink every day: A daily beer will add 15 pounds in a year, and one "hard" drink each day adds 17 pounds.

Is wine a healthier option? You may have heard that a glass or two of red wine a day can increase your good (HDL) cholesterol and thus decrease your risk of heart disease. At 90 calories a glass, wine is less of a problem than beer, but a glass of wine a day will add nine pounds to your body by the end of the year. Mixed drinks provide no escape either: One piña colada per day will pack an extra 27 pounds on your body in a year!

There's another reason to avoid alcoholic beverages or cut way back on your consumption of them: Alcohol "dissolves" your inhibitions and "dilutes" your judgment, so you often end up eating the wrong foods and consuming larger portions when you've been drinking (just one small handful of peanuts contains 170 calories, of which 74 percent come from fat). After only one or two drinks, you lose the normal inhibitions that keep you from reaching for those nuts, and before you know it, you've gone through several handfuls. Let's face it: When you're drinking, you're simply not as careful about what you eat.

Am I telling you not to drink? No, but I want to make it very clear: When your goal is to lose weight and keep it off, the less alcohol you consume, the more likely you are to succeed.

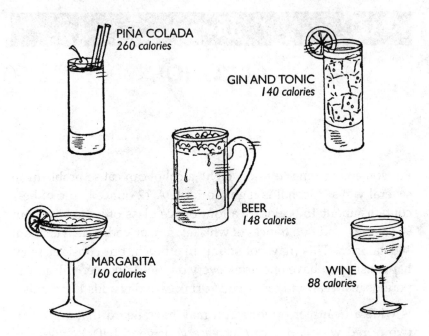

Because alcohol contains plenty of calories, it can cause problems with your weight-loss program. As the illustration shows, the caloric content varies among different types of drinks, so choose alcoholic beverages carefully. By making thoughtful selections, and cutting back your overall intake, even small changes can make a big difference over time.

DAY 20

Assignment

1. Decrease fat in your diet so it accounts for less than 20 percent of your total calories for the day. To accomplish this, increase your intake of foods that have 10 percent or less of their calories from fat and cut back significantly on foods with 30 percent or more of their calories from fat.

2. Cover 10,000 feet (walking or running at any pace, continuously or in smaller segments).

3. Walk up three flights of stairs.

4. Eat your meals using the pacing system, pausing 30 seconds between each bite.

5. Eat at least three meals.

6. Choose one of the following:

   a. Instead of an alcoholic beverage, try a fruit juice spritzer (for example, half cranberry juice and half seltzer water). Any bartender can easily make this drink for you.

   b. Get out of your beverage rut today—try a new, exotic fruit juice, a mango-flavored iced tea, or a cappuccino (use non-fat milk and hold the whipped cream).

7. Using your Self-Monitoring tearout chart, score yourself at the end of the day for goals accomplished.

DAY 21

PLATEAUS

Almost everyone who tries to lose weight gets stuck once in a while. Even though you continue doing everything in exactly the same way, your weight stabilizes for several days. As frustrating as these plateaus can be, you shouldn't let them upset you. In nearly all cases, a plateau is merely a sign that you're retaining water. Even though your weight isn't going down, if you are sticking closely to your plan, you are still continuing to burn fat.

Some weight-loss programs recommend trying to exercise yourself through a plateau. But weight plateaus are a complicated phenomenon, and generally physical activity alone does not remedy the situation. In fact, some people actually retain water when they start an exercise program, and the initial result may be a brief increase in weight. What's more, if you overdo exercise—as you may tend to do when you are feeling frustrated or upset about your weight—you run the risk of injuring yourself.

The best advice when you reach a weight plateau is to be patient. Bide your time. A plateau should be viewed as a temporary situation. Stick to your plan—continue to eat low-fat food, adjust your eating behavior, and get regular moderate exercise—and you will eventually get past the plateau.

DAY 21

Assignment

1. Decrease fat in your diet so it accounts for less than 20 percent of your total calories for the day. To accomplish this, increase your intake of foods that have 10 percent or less of their calories from fat and cut back significantly on foods with 30 percent or more of their calories from fat.

2. Cover 10,500 feet (walking or running at any pace, continuously or in smaller segments).

3. Walk up three flights of stairs.

4. Eat your meals using the pacing system, pausing 30 seconds between each bite.

5. Eat at least three meals.

6. Using your Self-Monitoring tearout chart, score yourself at the end of the day for goals accomplished.

7. Review this week's progress on your chart. Are you having a difficult time accomplishing your daily goals? Is one area (decreasing fat, increasing physical activity, pacing your eating, or monitoring) more difficult than another for you? Analyze your strengths and weaknesses, and develop a strategy for overcoming any problems in your way.

8. Weigh yourself today.

DAY 22

SNACKING

Eating three meals a day is a way of life for most Americans—not in response to any basic bodily need, but as a result of social convention. Nevertheless, there are bound to be times when you get hungry between meals. Many diets advise against eating between meals and suggest that by snacking you are somehow cheating. These diets are setting you up for failure. Your hunger drive is a powerful one and, should you try to fight it, you will almost certainly lose.

In this program, snacking is encouraged—but only if you are really hungry. If you don't eat when your body tells you it's hungry, you'll find yourself in an uphill battle. The more you deny yourself, the hungrier you'll get and the harder it will be not to eat. When you finally do give in, chances are you'll gorge yourself—often on highly fattening foods.

Although you cannot consciously turn off the hunger signal, you need not let your body dictate what you feed it. Just because your body is signaling you to eat cookies doesn't mean that it won't be satisfied with fresh fruit. When true hunger is the issue, fruit will be satisfying. When it's stress that is prompting you to eat, neither fruit nor cookies will ease that stress.

When you do decide to snack, use the same principles as at mealtime. First, choose foods that are low in fat. You may find this a little more difficult, given the fact that most typical snack foods (like chips and cookies) are very high in fat. There are, however, simple ways to create delicious, low-fat snacks. Here are a few examples:

Substitute fresh vegetables and salsa for potato chips and dip or for tortilla chips and guacamole. A one-ounce portion of chips and two tablespoons of dip contain 127 calories from fat, while a comparable serving of veggies and salsa contain virtually none. By making this change once a week over the course of a year, you'll save 6,604 fat calories—or nearly two pounds.

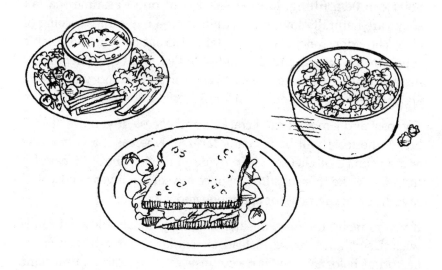

Snacking doesn't have to undermine your weight-loss efforts. There are many nonfat or low-fat choices in snacks and sandwiches, and they can contribute to an overall fat-reduction plan.

If you must have chips, try a fat-free or low-fat variety. Baked tortilla chips, for example, have only nine fat calories per one-ounce serving, compared to more than 50 in the fried variety. Make this change once a week for a year and you'll keep half a pound of fat off your body.

Select non-fat yogurt instead of regular. An eight-ounce container of non-fat yogurt contains less than five fat calories, while regular yogurt has close to 25. Make this substitution twice a week for a year and save yourself close to two pounds worth of fat calories (5,720 fat calories).

Stock your freezer with frozen sorbet bars (0 fat calories per bar) rather than ice cream (124 fat calories for a typical bar). Substitute sorbet for ice cream twice a week for a year and you'll save 12,896 fat calories—or close to three pounds.

Next time you find yourself reaching for the cookie jar, try a piece of fresh fruit instead. Two cream-filled chocolate cookies contain 44 fat calories; an apple contains only four. Do this twice a week for a year and save over a pound in fat calories (4,160).

Soup can be a filling, low-fat snack, but don't assume that all soups are naturally low in fat. A nine-and-a half-ounce serving of clam chowder, for instance, contains 135 fat calories. Vegetable soup, on the other hand, has only 36. Pick the vegetable variety instead of the chowder once a week for a year and you'll save about one and a half pounds in fat (5,148 fat calories).

Try toast and jam instead of crackers and cheese. If you use "light" bread, the toast will be virtually fat-free, whereas a few crackers and an ounce of cheese will provide you with about 95 calories from fat. Make this substitution once a week for a year and you'll save 4,940 fat calories—or about one and a half pounds.

If you're really hungry, consider making yourself a low-fat sandwich. Use "light" bread instead of regular; fat-free turkey slices instead of bologna; non-fat cheese instead of regular; and mustard instead of mayonnaise—and you can reduce the number of fat calories by over 250. Make that change once a week for a year and you'll save 13,260 fat calories or almost four pounds. (Add condiments like tomato, onion, and hot peppers to your heart's content. They're naturally low in fat and will add flavor and volume to your sandwich.)

Another important rule of thumb to follow when snacking: Eat slowly. All too often, people snack without thinking. They nibble on cookies while they work or put away a bowl of ice cream in front of the television. Snacking like this is a sure way to overeat. It causes you to eat too fast, so you don't recognize that you are full until too late. Just as important—because you're not paying attention, you'll draw little pleasure from the taste and feel of your food. As a result, it will take more food to satisfy you.

To help slow yourself down, make it a rule never to snack while doing something else. A good way to carry this out is by forcing yourself to snack only at the dining table (leaving all distractions, like magazines and newspapers, well out of reach). Concentrate fully on the food you are eating and, just as you do at mealtime, wait 30 seconds between bites. If you're forced to eat at work, at least stop your work while eating. Clear your desk and focus on your food—you'll enjoy it more and eat less.

DAY 22

Assignment

1. Decrease fat in your diet so it accounts for less than 20 percent of your total calories for the day. To accomplish this, increase your intake of foods that have 10 percent or less of their calories from fat and cut back significantly on foods with 30 percent or more of their calories from fat.

2. Cover 11,000 feet (walking or running at any pace, continuously or in smaller segments).

3. Walk up four flights of stairs.

4. Eat your meals using the pacing system, pausing 30 seconds between each bite.

5. Eat at least three meals.

6. Choose one of the following:

   a. Go to the market and stock up on low-fat or nonfat snack items so you'll have them available at home, at work, and when you go out. Having such snacks handy will help you make good food choices when you are hungry. For example, always have a favorite fruit (apples, bananas, and oranges travel especially well) or some vegetables in your purse, briefcase, or car for a ready snack (wrap the vegetables well, and you won't have to worry about the moisture).

   b. Try a carmel-flavored rice cake or a frozen fruit bar today to satisfy your craving for a sweet snack.

7. Using your Self-Monitoring tearout chart, score yourself at the end of the day for goals accomplished.

DAY 23

BODY FAT

If you are obsessed with the number on the bathroom scale, your attention is focused on the wrong number. Your body fat percentage is more important, because the composition of your body influences your health much more than your absolute weight.

Your body fat percentage tells you what proportion of your weight is composed of fat and what percentage comes from lean tissues (muscle, bone, and other vital organs). As this body fat percentage rises, you have a greater chance of developing chronic diseases such as high blood pressure, heart disease, and diabetes.

The "ideal" body percentage differs between men and women. Men should try to maintain their body fat at no more than 20 percent; women should aim for 30 percent or less. In the past, many experts believed that your body fat percentage could rise as you aged and still stay within acceptable parameters—up to 25 percent for men, and 35 percent for women. However, recent studies have shown that no matter how old you are, you should try to keep your body fat at or under the lower (20 and 30 percent) figures.

At the other extreme, your body fat percentage can become too low. Women who fall below 20 percent body fat often find that their menstrual periods stop; at even lower fat levels, they may experience bone loss, making them susceptible to a bone thinning disease called osteoporosis. For men, the risk of medical complications begins to rise when body fat goes below 12 percent. Leaner isn't always better and could even pose health risks in some cases.

Some people—particularly those who are physically inactive—have relatively normal scale weight but lots of excess body fat. Other individuals might be considered "heavy" by standard tables, but much of their weight is made up of muscle, so it's actually quite acceptable.

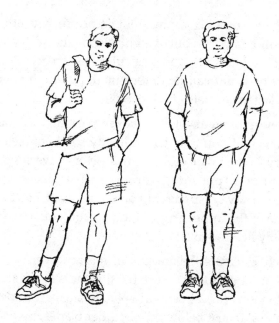

Here are two men, each weighing 200 pounds. The first man's body fat is 20 percent, and thus 200 pounds is his ideal weight. However, at 30 percent, the second man has too much body fat, and should work to cut his body-fat percentage.

What's the best way to measure your body fat percentage? The bathroom scale won't help, since it can't tell you how much of your body weight is fat and how much is muscle or lean tissue. Instead, choose from one of the following techniques for an evaluation of your body composition:

Underwater weighing. For many years, this method (also called hydrodensitometry) has been the gold standard for measuring body density and the percentage of body fat. In this procedure, you are completely immersed in a tank of water while sitting on an underwater scale. You are instructed to expel as much air as possible from your lungs while underwater, and then your underwater weight is measured. Since fat is less dense and more buoyant than bone, muscle, and organ tissue, everyone will weigh less underwater than out of the water. The greater proportion of body fat you have, the more buoyant you will be, the less you will weigh in the water tank, and the greater the difference will be between your weights in and out of the water.

Once you have surfaced, a physiologist or other health-care professional will compare your weight out of the water with your underwater weight. With a few calculations, an accurate percentage of total body fat can be determined, although some of that accuracy is lost in severely obese people.

Skin-fold measurement. This is the simplest and least expensive test—and one that you may have already tried yourself in a very rudimentary fashion. For years, some doctors have suggested that people perform a "pinch test" on themselves, using thumb and forefinger to firmly grasp the skin on their side at waist level or on the backside of the upper arm. If they pinched more than an inch, they probably had too much body fat.

To accurately calculate the amount of fat, however, it's necessary to use special calipers to measure the thickness of the skin fold (or the subcutaneous fat) at several specific sites around the body, including the skin just below the shoulder blades, over the triceps muscle, on the skin of the abdomen (at the waistline), and over the front of the thigh. The sum of these measurements (in millimeters) is used to calculate your body fat percentage. Some health clubs and fitness centers have the correct calipers and trained personnel who can perform these measurements accurately.

While skin-fold measurements are fairly reliable for the average person, the calipers must be placed at exactly the same spots on the skin each time to measure changes.

Accu-Measure. One fairly accurate way to check body fat yourself is with a device called Accu-Measure, which can be purchased for about $20. It might be described as a sophisticated, do-it-yourself pinch test, utilizing specially designed plastic calipers to grasp and measure a fold of fat. Using this measurement and the numerical tables that come with the device, you can calculate your body fat percentage. The high price of these calipers can be at least partially justified by the clever design which makes the results more reliable and reproducible. With this device, you'll actually be able to see the changes in your body fat percentage as your weight drops. The device can be ordered by phone (1-800-866-2727).

Bioelectrical impedance analysis. This technique determines body composition by evaluating how the body reacts to an electrical current transmitted through it. Electrodes (just like those used for an electrocardiogram) are attached to the body, usually at the hand and the foot. Then a harmless electrical current is passed through you (don't worry—the current is so mild you can't even feel it). The current is conducted more easily through lean muscle mass (which has a higher water content), while fat tends to impede it. So, the more muscle tissue you have in relation to fat, the faster the current moves through your body. A computer evaluates the rate of electrical flow and calculates the body fat percentage from this information.

Bioelectrical impedance analysis is not a perfect test, however, and is considered less reliable than underwater weighing. A recent study concluded that the findings of this test can be undermined by an individual's body shape, skin moisture, what he or she has eaten or drank in the hours preceding the test, and even the close proximity of electrical appliances.

DEXA. A new technology called dual-energy x-ray absorptiometry (DEXA) is another alternative for measuring body fat. It involves taking a total body scan, which can measure not only fat, but also bone and muscle density. This same technology is used to monitor bone loss in women with osteoporosis, and while it exposes you to some radiation, the doses are extremely low—much lower than a routine x-ray. Since DEXA scanning does involve some radiation exposure, however, it's not a test you would use frequently to track your progress; calipers and underwater weighing are better for this purpose. The DEXA procedure takes about 30 minutes and costs approximately $150 but is not yet widely available.

No matter what method you choose to measure your body fat percentage, you can use the information to help set goals for yourself. Over time, you want to reduce your body fat levels until they are in line with the ideal percentages mentioned earlier. The strategies that form the basis for this book—including low-fat eating and regular exercise—will help achieve that goal.

DAY 23

Assignment

1. Decrease fat in your diet so it accounts for less than 20 percent of your total calories for the day. To accomplish this, increase your intake of foods that have 10 percent or less of their calories from fat and cut back significantly on foods with 30 percent or more of their calories from fat.

2. Cover 11,500 feet (walking or running at any pace, continuously or in smaller segments).

3. Walk up four flights of stairs.

4. Eat your meals using the pacing system, pausing 30 seconds between each bite.

5. Eat at least three meals.

6. Choose one of the following:

    a. If you want to measure your body fat without investing a lot of money, call your local health club or hospital to see if they offer this service for a nominal fee. They often have high-quality calipers and trained personnel available for this purpose.

    b. Try some of the strength training exercises in this book (see pages 99-104).

7. Using your Self-Monitoring tearout chart, score yourself at the end of the day for goals accomplished.

DAY 24

WHAT TO DO WHEN YOUR WEIGHT REGULATOR FIGHTS BACK

As you near the end of the 28-day Conditioning Phase, you may notice a subtle slowing in the rate at which you are losing weight (people with only a few pounds to lose may have noticed it earlier). Weight that came off easily in the first few weeks of the program starts coming off more slowly, even though you're still completing all of the daily assignments to the letter.

Don't get frustrated—this slowdown is to be expected. It's your weight regulator's last ditch attempt to maintain its abnormal set point and prevent you from losing more weight. Your weight-regulating system has a built-in mechanism for slowing your weight-loss efforts: It changes your metabolic rate (remember, that's the baseline rate at which your body burns calories while you're at rest). When weight is being lost, the weight regulator tries to slow the process by causing your body to burn fewer calories. When weight is being gained, just the opposite occurs: The weight regulator speeds up your baseline metabolism, causing you to burn more calories throughout the day (and night).

A recent study at Rockefeller University illustrates this phenomenon quite nicely. Researchers measured the amount of calories burned during a 24-hour period by a group of 41 men and women. Some of these people were then intentionally underfed until they lost 10 percent of their initial body weight; others were overfed until they gained 10 percent of their starting weight. The investigators then remeasured the number of calories these people burned in 24 hours. The group who lost weight burned an average of 15 percent fewer calories, while those who put on weight burned 16 percent more.

In simple English, this means that as you lose weight, your body makes you work a little harder to lose each subsequent pound. It does *not* mean that you won't be able to lose more weight by doing the same things that worked at first. You'll just have to accept a slower rate of weight loss. Don't get discouraged. Your metabolic rate will never slow down enough to completely negate your continued efforts to lose weight, just as when you overeat it never speeds up enough to burn up all the extra calories.

When your rate of weight loss begins to slow, it's tempting to try things that could speed it up again. For example, some people try to overpower their weight regulator by cutting back dramatically on their food intake or greatly increasing their exercise level. *Please* don't make these mistakes. Cutting way back on your calories will speed your weight loss temporarily, but it accomplishes this by destroying lean muscle tissues, not by depleting the body fat you've stored. And rapidly increasing the amount of exercise you do will produce only modest changes in weight loss, while significantly increasing your risk of injuries. Before you try these potentially dangerous methods, remember that accepting gradual weight loss is a key factor for success over the long term. Be patient with the steady weight loss that occurs when you stick to our plan, and you will ultimately reach your final goal.

DAY 24

Assignment

1. Decrease fat in your diet so it accounts for less than 20 percent of your total calories for the day. To accomplish this, increase your intake of foods that have 10 percent or less of their calories from fat and cut back significantly on foods with 30 percent or more of their calories from fat.

2. Cover 12,000 feet (walking or running at any pace, continuously or in smaller segments).

3. Walk up four flights of stairs.

4. Eat your meals using the pacing system, pausing 30 seconds between each bite.

5. Eat at least three meals.

6. Choose one of the following:

   a. Today, try a different time of day for all or part of your walk. You'll be surprised to see how much the surroundings change. Varying the time of day is a good way to keep your walks interesting.

   b. Reward yourself today for following the program. Rent a movie you've been wanting to see or go to a play or a sporting event with a friend.

7. Using your Self-Monitoring tearout chart, score yourself at the end of the day for goals accomplished.

DAY 25

BANKING CALORIES

Once a year—on my birthday—I make reservations at the best steakhouse in Los Angeles for a dinner that breaks all the rules. You should see the stares I get from people around me as I polish off my own 16-ounce porterhouse steak and then feast on everyone else's leftovers. Why do I do this? Because I love the taste of steak, so I indulge myself once a year in a big way. How do I get away with it? By "banking" calories ahead of time.

Every year, eight or nine days before my birthday, I start shaving about 100 additional fat calories off what I normally eat each day. I literally "bank" those fat calories, and by the time my birthday arrives, I've established nearly 1,000 "calorie credits." That's more than enough fat calories to compensate for the fat in the steak, so I'm able to enjoy my meal guilt-free. The morning after my birthday, I feel great knowing there's nothing to "pay" for—except the dinner bill.

I'm sure you have times that call for indulging, too, like your birthday, your anniversary, or a romantic evening on your Hawaiian vacation. So indulge yourself. You just have to learn *how* to do it without losing too much ground on your weight-loss program. The key to success is planning ahead.

Before the "big event" arrives, estimate the number of fat calories you expect to consume. Then start setting aside or "banking" those fat calories ahead of time. Since a gram of fat contains more than twice the number of calories than either a gram of carbohydrate or a gram of protein, banking fat calories minimizes the cutbacks you have to make to achieve your goal. If your goal is to bank 100 calories a day, for instance, eliminating just one slice of cheese a day (which gets most of its calories from fat) would be enough. If, however, you tried to save the calories by cutting back on a low-fat food like fat-free luncheon meat, you'd have to give up nearly three ounces of food to bank the same number of calories.

Don't make the mistake of trying to bank too many calories in one day. Somewhere between 100 and 150 calories a day is a reasonable goal. By trying to cut back more than that, your nutrition is bound to suffer.

Calorie banking can also be used to help you recover from an occasional unexpected overindulgence (we're only human). In this case, you'll be slowly paying back the fat calories you "borrowed," instead of building up a credit ahead of time. This gradual payback is much safer and more effective over the long run than skipping entire meals or fasting (as so many people do to make up for deviating from their plan).

However, calorie banking should be used only for special occasions, not as a way to avoid your regular plan. People who overuse this process have great difficulty losing weight. When they're not overindulging themselves, they're banking calories for the next opportunity they get to overindulge. So, don't let calorie-banking become a way of life. When used properly, it's a great tool for enjoying life while staying on track with your weight-loss plan.

DAY 25

Assignment

1. Decrease fat in your diet so it accounts for less than 20 percent of your total calories for the day. To accomplish this, increase your intake of foods that have 10 percent or less of their calories from fat and cut back significantly on foods with 30 percent or more of their calories from fat.

2. Cover 12,500 feet (walking or running at any pace, continuously or in smaller segments).

3. Walk up four flights of stairs.

4. Eat your meals using the pacing system, pausing 30 seconds between each bite.

5. Eat at least three meals.

6. Choose one of the following:

   a. In addition to your walking assignment today, try a new physical activity. For example, go bowling, play a round of miniature golf, or go on a nature hike.

   b. Try a different low-fat or nonfat salad dressing (either one you bought or one you made yourself). So many choices are available that you'll want to experiment to find one or two you really like.

7. Using your Self-Monitoring tearout chart, score yourself at the end of the day for goals accomplished.

DAY 26

FAST FOOD

Those omnipresent drive-through lanes at America's fast-food restaurants can be hazardous to your health—and to your weight-loss goals. Yes, fast-food outlets are convenient and economical, and they complement the fast-paced lifestyles of many people. But most of their menu items are brimming with fat.

Just consider a report published in the *New England Journal of Medicine*, which estimated that in the typical fast food meal, 40 to 55 percent of calories come from fat. A single deluxe cheeseburger and an order of fries can sabotage the rest of your day's efforts at weight control.

Fortunately, some fast-food chains are getting the message that many Americans are fed up with high-fat foods. And because these restaurants are unwilling to sacrifice such a large share of their potential market, they are now providing at least some low-fat choices.

What should you look for when you walk through the golden arches or one of its competitors? Here are a few of the healthier options:

- Go for salad bars. Choose fresh greens like lettuce and spinach, and then add lots of vegetables and fruit (like mushrooms, carrots, cauliflower, peppers, onions, pineapples, and tomatoes), and a low-calorie dressing or lemon juice. Stay away from coleslaw, potato salad, macaroni salad, nuts, avocado, and eggs. And don't overdo it with high-fat toppings like bacon bits, olives, and shredded cheese. If you like their flavor, sprinkle them very lightly over your salad—lightly enough so you can still enjoy the flavor of the vegetables.

- Forget the French fries, and choose a baked potato instead. But be careful about what you put on top. Eating potatoes plain makes the most sense (many people laugh at this idea, but once they've tasted the real flavor of an unspoiled potato, they never use as much topping again). If plain potatoes don't appeal to you, try toppings such as onions or salsa. Avoid cheese (it's probably a high-fat variety), sour cream, chili, and bacon bits, or use them very sparingly—just enough to get their taste.

- If you're yearning for a hamburger, choose one of the leaner varieties. McDonald's McLean burger gets 28 percent of its calories from fat, which is much more acceptable than the 49 percent fat calories in a Big Mac. Or choose a regular burger instead of one with two patties and cheese, and request it with mustard or ketchup, onions, and tomatoes, but without the "special sauce."

- At a pizza parlor, order your pizza without cheese (or with less cheese), and ask for extra tomato sauce and healthy toppings—including green peppers, onions, mushrooms, tomatoes, and pineapple. Stay away from toppings such as sausage and pepperoni.

- For drinks, choose water, iced tea, nonfat milk, orange juice, or diet sodas rather than milk shakes or regular soft drinks.

- Some menu items might seem like good choices because of their names—but don't be fooled. For example, chicken or fish sandwiches sound healthier than hamburgers—but they may be even higher in fat and calories. In most cases, they're breaded and fried, which instantly elevates them from a low- to a high-fat entree. A better choice: a chicken fajita, although you may have to special-order it to ensure that it's not bathed in oil, sour cream, and guacamole; ask for extra vegetables and salsa instead.

- If you're having breakfast at a fast-food chain, avoid (except very occasionally) breakfast sandwiches, which usually are filled with cheese, egg, and sausage. Hotcakes with syrup are a better alternative, as is cereal with nonfat or low-fat milk.

DAY 26

Assignment

1. Decrease fat in your diet so it accounts for less than 20 percent of your total calories for the day. To accomplish this, increase your intake of foods that have 10 percent or less of their calories from fat and cut back significantly on foods with 30 percent or more of their calories from fat.

2. Cover 13,000 feet (walking or running at any pace, continuously or in smaller segments).

3. Walk up four flights of stairs.

4. Eat your meals using the pacing system, pausing 30 seconds between each bite.

5. Eat at least three meals.

6. Choose one of the following:

   a. At your favorite fast-food restaurant, try the "light" version of your favorite food.

   b. Customize your fast-food order to reduce fat. For example, hold the cheese, mayonnaise, and "special sauce" on your sandwich, opting for ketchup, mustard, tomato, and onions instead.

7. Using your Self-Monitoring tearout chart, score yourself at the end of the day for goals accomplished.

DAY 27

FIVE MORE WAYS TO DECREASE FAT

It's easy to come up with ways to dramatically reduce the amount of fat in your diet: Stop eating all desserts and meats, to name just two. However, these types of sweeping changes are difficult—if not impossible—for most people to make. Some may succeed for short periods of time, but very few people can live with such radical dietary changes over the long term.

Fortunately, there is an easier way: Make smaller, less noticeable reductions in fat. In other words, make changes you can live with. There are an endless number of clever ways to cut small amounts of fat from your diet. Here are just a few:

1. Reduce Your Serving Size. Most people hate the idea of having to eat less. But the fact is, even a tiny reduction in the size of your portions helps. Just leaving a few bites behind at every meal, for example, adds up over time. If done consistently, these few bites can amount to several pounds of fat over the course of a year.

Try serving yourself a little less than you usually eat. However, don't make the mistake of cutting back too drastically. Cut back by only 10 percent or so. A good way to do this is to serve yourself as you normally would and then put a little bit back into the serving dish.

Also, don't feel you need to cut back on everything. Concentrate on the high-fat dishes and don't worry about those that are low in fat. In fact, you may want to increase your serving size of low-fat foods in order to compensate for the reductions you're making elsewhere. Filling up on a side dish of steamed vegetables, for example, will allow you to cut back on a high-fat main dish and still leave the table feeling satisfied.

Here are two examples of how small reductions can add up over a period of time:

Eat one-and-a-half pieces of pizza instead of two and save 68 fat calories. Make this change twice a month for one year and you'll save yourself about half a pound of fat (1,768 fat calories).

Have half a slice of Swiss cheese instead of a full slice and save 37 fat calories. Do it twice a week for a year and save a pound of fat (3,848 fat calories).

2. Pick the Brand with the Least Fat. Do you reach for the same brands every time you shop for groceries? Most of us do. We find a brand we like and stick with it, sometimes because we like the taste; other times because it costs less. But different brands of the same food product can vary dramatically in the amount of fat they contain.

The only way to determine which brand is lowest in fat is by reading the labels and comparing. Next time you shop for groceries, compare each of your favorite brands to three or four others. If yours is lower in fat than most, go ahead and buy it; if it's comparatively high in fat, give one of the other brands a try (you can always switch back if you don't like it). For a few examples of how switching brands can cut your fat intake see the box on page 230.

3. Use "Reduced Fat," "Light," or "Fat-Free" Alternatives When They Are Available. The number of "reduced fat," "light," and "fat-free" products on the supermarket shelves has multiplied rapidly in the past several years. It seems that everything from potato chips to cheese to cookies to cakes is now available in a low-fat variety.

Although the best foods to eat when you're trying to lose weight are naturally low in fat (and therefore won't have a low-fat equivalent), when you are purchasing food that is usually relatively high in fat, look for a low-fat version of it. (See "Making Lower-Fat Choices," page 232.) In order to qualify as "reduced fat" a product must have at least 25 percent less fat per serving than the product it is being compared to. (For example, if regular potato chips contain 10 grams of fat per serving, the reduced chips can

FAT SAVINGS

Here are a few examples of the kinds of fat savings you can expect:

SMOKED TURKEY SLICES (2 OZ.)

Butterball	*22 fat calories*
Healthy Deli	*10 fat calories*
Louis Rich	*7 fat calories*
Oscar Mayer	*5 fat calories*

Difference between highest and lowest: 17 fat calories

MICROWAVE POPCORN (3 CUPS)

Jiffy Pop	*46 fat calories*
Jolly Time	*58 fat calories*
Orville Redenbacher	*51 fat calories*
Pillsbury	*118 fat calories*
Planter's	*78 fat calories*

Difference between highest and lowest: 72 fat calories

MINESTRONE SOUP (9.5 OZ.)

Campbell's	*37 fat calories*
Healthy Choice	*22 fat calories*
Hormel	*11 fat calories*
Progresso	*31 fat calories*

Difference between highest and lowest: 26 fat calories

contain only 7.5.) Read labels carefully to make sure you're really getting a low-fat (and low-calorie) product.

Foods "light" in fat ("light" can also refer to a product's caloric or salt content) contain no more than half the fat of the original product. Products that are "fat-free" are even better—they contain virtually no fat whatsoever.

4. Never Add Fat to Your Food Once It's Been Prepared. It's easy to turn a low-fat dish into a high-fat one simply by adding lots of fat at the table. Pancakes, for instance, are very low in fat unless they've been smothered in butter, and many pasta dishes are low in fat until they get doused in Parmesan cheese.

Avoid adding fat—in any form—to your food once it has been prepared. Although you may initially miss the flavor that fat adds, you will quickly get used to it. Eventually, you won't be able to eat any other way.

If your food needs a lift when it gets to the table, try using low-fat items to jazz it up. For example, use jams and jellies instead of butter on pancakes and bread, or salsa instead of sour cream on baked potatoes. In some cases, actually adding small amounts of fat while preparing food will prevent you from adding much larger amounts at the table. If you just can't do without Parmesan cheese on your pasta, for example, adding a little to the sauce will lend the flavor of cheese to the dish and make it unnecessary to add more to your individual portion.

Some of the most common high-fat items used to dress up prepared foods include butter, sour cream, mayonnaise, and cheese. But you should rethink every "additive" you use:

- Putting two tablespoons of sour cream on a baked potato adds 52 fat calories. (Switching to two tablespoons of salsa saves virtually all of them.)

- For every tablespoon of Parmesan cheese used to flavor pasta, you add 22 fat calories.

- One pat of butter on toast contributes 35 calories, all of them from fat.

- One tablespoon of mayonnaise on a hamburger raises the number of fat calories by 100.

5. Reduce the Amount of Fat in Your Recipes. Most recipes call for much more fat than is necessary. In fact, you can cut the amount of fat in most recipes (except for those already designed to be low in fat) by one-third to one-half and not really notice a difference.

Butter and oil are the most obvious things you can cut back on. But other high-fat items like cheese and meat can be reduced as well.

- If a recipe calls for a half a cup of oil, add only two-thirds that amount and save over 650 calories in the dish.

- Use only ⅔ cup of grated cheese in a recipe that calls for a cup and save about 205 fat calories.

- Substitute one pound of extra-lean ground beef for one pound of regular ground beef in a recipe and save 390 fat calories.

When you reduce the amount of fat in a recipe, you may need to use nonstick cookware or a small amount of nonstick spray to prevent the food from sticking to the pan. You may also have to reduce your baking time, as low-fat baked goods tend to cook more quickly.

MAKING LOWER-FAT CHOICES

Here are a few examples of just how significant your fat savings can be:

Mayonnaise	*100 fat calories/tbsp.*
"Lite" Mayonnaise	*46 fat calories/tbsp.*
Microwave Popcorn	*58 fat calories/serving*
"Lite" Microwave Popcorn	*14 fat calories/serving*
Fruit-filled Cookies	*14 fat calories/cookie*
"Fat-free" Fruit-filled Cookies	*0 fat calories/cookie*
Italian Salad Dressing	*54 fat calories/tbsp.*
"Fat-free" Italian Salad Dressing	*0 fat calories/tbsp.*

DAY 27

Assignment

1. Decrease fat in your diet so it accounts for less than 20 percent of your total calories for the day. To accomplish this, increase your intake of foods that have 10 percent or less of their calories from fat and cut back significantly on foods with 30 percent or more of their calories from fat.

2. Cover 13,500 feet (walking or running at any pace, continuously or in smaller segments).

3. Walk up four flights of stairs.

4. Eat your meals using the pacing system, pausing 30 seconds between each bite.

5. Eat at least three meals.

6. Choose one of the following:

   a. When you serve your portions today, try to cut the initial amount you put on your plate. You'll be surprised to discover that one slice of bread is often as satisfying as two; a cup of soup is just as good as a bowl; two slices of lunch meat fill a sandwich as well as three. Give it a try.

   b. If you have not yet tried the low-fat or nonfat version of a particular food you like, try it today.

7. Using your Self-Monitoring tearout chart, score yourself at the end of the day for goals accomplished.

DAY 28

CONTINUATION OR MAINTENANCE?

This is the last day of the 28-day conditioning program, and most of the changes you've been making to lose weight should be starting to feel natural to you. Soon, low-fat foods will actually taste better than the high-fat dishes you were used to. You'll be the last one to finish at the dinner table. You'll even look forward to exercise.

If you didn't have much weight to lose when you started and you have already reached your final goal, you will now move on to the Maintenance Phase of our program (page 310). This phase is specifically designed to help you maintain the new weight level you have achieved while further improving your level of fitness.

If you still have more weight to lose, you will move on to the Continuity Phase of our program (page 241). This phase is designed to promote ongoing weight loss at a steady rate for as long as is necessary to take you to your final goal. The Continuity Phase of the program is based on the same scientific principles as the Conditioning Phase, but the activities and assignments have been modified to reflect the changes that are taking place in your body at this time.

The following questionnaire will help you define some special issues that you should be aware of before starting either the Continuity or Maintenance phases. Write your answers directly on the questionnaire; then use the Scorecard (page 236) to interpret your responses. From time to time, return to this questionnaire and check to see if your responses have changed. You should see progress each time you ask yourself these questions.

SELF-ASSESSMENT QUESTIONNAIRE

1. Compare your present sense of control over food with the control you had over food before you started this program.

0   1   2   3   4   5   6   7   8   9   10

LESS NOW   SAME   MORE NOW

2. Compare the nutritional quality of your diet now to the food you ate before you started this program.

0   1   2   3   4   5   6   7   8   9   10

WORSE NOW   SAME   BETTER NOW

3. Compare the amount of eating-related guilt you have now to the amount you experienced before starting this program.

0   1   2   3   4   5   6   7   8   9   10

MORE NOW   SAME   LESS NOW

4. Compare your overall fitness level now to your fitness level before starting this program.

0   1   2   3   4   5   6   7   8   9   10

WORSE NOW   SAME   BETTER NOW

5. Compare your energy level now to the way you felt before starting this program.

0   1   2   3   4   5   6   7   8   9   10

LOWER NOW   SAME   HIGHER NOW

6. When you started this program, what was the ultimate goal you wanted to reach? _____ POUNDS

7. What is the ultimate goal you want to reach now? _____POUNDS

8. How much weight have you lost in the past 28 days? _____POUNDS

9. How much weight do you want to lose in the next 28 days? _____POUNDS

10. At this point in the program, how would you rate your weight-loss efforts?

0   1   2   3   4   5   6   7   8   9   10

FAILURE   SUCCESS

SCORECARD

Question 1: Research shows that people who *feel* in control are more successful at losing weight and keeping it off than people who don't feel this way. In part, it's like a self-fulfilling prophecy: If you believe you can be successful at something, you're more likely to be successful at it. But it's not just wishful thinking, and it's not a placebo effect. There are many skills you can learn that actually *do* increase your control.

During the Conditioning Phase of our program, you learned many of these skills. The low-fat assignments taught you how to control the foods you eat; the exercise assignments taught you how to control your schedule and strengthened your control over the natural tendency to resist exercise; and the pacing program showed you how to control the subconscious eating urges that make you consume food even when you aren't hungry.

Whether you have more weight to lose or not, it is important that you continue to practice these skills until they become absolutely second nature to you. Once that happens, you should be able to control your weight without great effort or sacrifice. You will also be able to enjoy the additional benefit of *feeling* more in control of your life.

Question 2: Unless you were on a very low-fat diet before you started our program, the overall nutritional quality of your food intake has probably improved significantly since you started our program. That's because changing from high-fat foods to low-fat choices almost automatically increases your intake of vitamins, minerals, fiber, and complex carbohydrates.

As you enter the next phase of this program, it's very helpful to recognize this additional benefit of a low-fat diet. In fact, it's a good idea to select foods as much because they are nutritious as for their low-fat content (the two features generally go hand-in-hand). Emphasizing these nutritional benefits will not only strengthen your resolve to choose good foods in the supermarket, it may also make you feel better generally (this *is* a placebo effect, but who cares).

Question 3: Probably no other emotion is associated with body weight more than guilt. Much of it is based on the now-outdated notion that obesity is the consequence of willful overeating or willful inactivity. As a result, overweight people are "blamed" for their condition, and made to feel guilty about it. The process starts during childhood, in the form of painful criticisms from probably well-meaning parents, and continues through adult life with hurtful jibes and accusatory glances from family, friends, coworkers, and even physicians.

The problem of guilt is made even worse by rigid diet plans, which set rules that cannot be followed, and then blame people who break the rules for being "weak-willed." But there is no place in any weight-loss program for guilt. It is neither appropriate nor productive. Indeed, it shifts your focus in the wrong direction and undermines whatever plan you are following.

So what do you do when you "slip" on our program if feeling guilty has always been your natural response? Blame me instead. After all, if this program were perfect, there wouldn't be any slips, would there? And after you get done blaming me, take a moment to learn from your slip. Identify the weakness in my program (as it applies in your particular case), and prepare a more effective strategy for dealing with the same issue the next time around. Reacting this way will not only relieve the guilt, but also reduce the number of guilt-provoking episodes that occur in the future.

Question 4: Many weight-loss programs actually decrease the fitness levels of their participants by cutting calories back too far. This caloric restriction causes muscle destruction and metabolic changes that reduce strength and decrease endurance. By promoting only modest caloric restriction and increases in your physical activity, our program is designed to achieve exactly the opposite .

If you've been doing all of our exercise assignments (or substituting equivalent activities), your fitness level should already be significantly higher. If you have not already noticed a change, take a little time to look for it. Subjectively, you may notice that you simply feel stronger and more energetic. But there are also some objective measures of fitness you can use to mark your progress. These include your heart rate during vigorous exercise, your recovery rate (the more fit you are, the more quickly your heart rate will return to normal after exercise), and your resting heart rate (mine is 52 beats per minute; you should check yours from time to time).

Question 5: Some people think that the more work they do, the more tired they should feel. But for people who are fit, added work is actually invigorating. If that sounds strange to you, compare the way you feel on the days you do our exercise assignments to the days you don't. If you've really been doing all of the exercise assignments (or substituting equivalent activities), you should be noting an increased energy level by now.

Question 6: Most people starting a weight-loss program have an "ultimate" goal in mind. But all too often, their goal is unrealistic—sometimes even inappropriate (usually much too low for their height and bone structure). That's the start of a losing battle, because that much weight loss not only jeopardizes their health, but makes their weight-regulating system even more resistant to their efforts.

Another problem with ultimate goals is that, all too often, they become the *only* goal—the sole definition of success. And, very frequently, people who become overly focused on their ultimate goals lose sight of the intermediate goals they are accomplishing along the way. Especially if they have large amounts of weight to lose, they fail to appreciate the accomplishments they have already made, they become discouraged more easily, and they give up entirely.

Question 7: Take a moment now to reevaluate the final goal you have set for yourself. If you have selected a goal that is lower than it should be, this is the time to set a new and more realistic goal. If you are not sure what your final goal should be, trust your body to find its own best weight as long too you eat well and remain active. And try not to focus too much on your final goal. Always make the next pound your most important goal, and the final goal will take care of itself.

Question 8: Most people who use our program experience their most rapid weight loss during the first 28 days. This occurs because they are making the greatest changes in diet and activity levels at this time, and also because it takes a while for their weight-regulating system to start resisting their efforts. As you look at the number of pounds you have lost during the first 28 days, it's important to recognize that you are not likely to continue losing at that rate.

Question 9: If you skipped ahead and read Chapter 11 already, you know the correct answer to this question is "four pounds." Why only four pounds? Because that is the starting goal I've established for everyone during the initial 28 days of our Continuity Phase. And that is the goal I want you to set for yourself during the next 28 days, even though it may be much lower than what you lost during the first 28. In Chapter 11, I'll explain why I picked this goal. In the meantime, I'd like you to start thinking of four pounds as your next goal (not necessarily your last goal). If you are discouraged by that goal for the next four weeks, read on. I think you'll change your mind after you learn why we picked it.

Question 10: If you answered this question with a "10," you earned a perfect score. If you circled anything lower than a "6," go back to the beginning of the book and start reading all over again, because you have missed the most important message that I have to give you, and that is: You are a success, no matter what your weight is, and you must stop thinking of this program in terms of success or failure. The fact is, you are trying new things, learning new skills and adding new information to your store of knowledge. It is not possible to fail when you are doing these things.

DAY 28

Assignment

1. Decrease fat in your diet so it accounts for less than 20 percent of your total calories for the day. To accomplish this, increase your intake of foods that have 10 percent or less of their calories from fat and cut back significantly on foods with 30 percent or more of their calories from fat.

2. Cover 14,000 feet (walking or running at any pace, continuously or in smaller segments).

3. Walk up four flights of stairs.

4. Eat your meals using the pacing system, pausing 30 seconds between each bite.

5. Eat at least three meals.

6. Using your Self-Monitoring tearout chart, score yourself at the end of the day for goals accomplished.

7. Review this week's progress on your chart. Are you having a difficult time accomplishing your daily goals? Is one area (decreasing fat, increasing physical activity, pacing your eating, or monitoring) more difficult than another for you? Analyze your strengths and weaknesses, and develop a strategy for overcoming any problems in your way.

11

TAKING IT OFF:
THE CONTINUITY PHASE

During the first 28 days, our program focused on four primary activities designed to promote weight loss and recondition the way your mind and body react to food and physical activity. After finishing this portion of the program, most people are surprised by how much weight they have lost during this four-week period, because the changes they made were so gradual and easy. Many are also surprised by how natural their new attitudes and behaviors feel after just 28 days. This contrasts greatly with the typical experiences most people have had with commercial weight-loss programs and diet plans, which produce (temporary) results through severe caloric restriction, rigid menu plans, high intensity exercise, and sheer willpower—and which leave people feeling deprived, abused, and ravenously hungry.

There is, however, one minor problem with our conditioning program: It cannot endlessly produce weight loss for you at the same rate you experienced during the first four weeks. That's because your weight regulator starts to fight back as soon as it recognizes that your weight has dropped significantly. At this point, you could fight back even harder, cutting more fat, adding more exercise, and slowing your eating even more—which risks your health, interferes with your joy of eating, and causes your weight regulator to fight back even harder. Or you can beat the regulator at its own game—continuing your basic activities, and being content with a slower rate of weight loss that your weight regulator won't fight as vigorously. This new phase of our program, the "Continuity Phase" is based on this latter, wiser course.

There is only one way to lose fat and protect muscle, and that is *slowly.* If you still have ten pounds to lose after the first 28 days, the Continuity Phase will help you lose it—slowly, but surely and steadily. If you are 100 pounds overweight, the Continuity Phase will just as surely and just as steadily help you lose that, too. The only difference will be the amount of time it takes to reach your goal.

If you have 100 pounds to lose (or even 40, 60, or 80), you may now be wondering if the same program that is right for someone with only ten pounds to lose is also right for you. You might also be tempted to turn to a program that promises drastic weight loss much more rapidly. That is precisely the kind of thinking that gets many people into trouble—by pushing them to try deficient and dangerous diets and weight-loss plans that promise rapid, massive weight loss, at any cost.

Please, don't let yourself make that mistake. If you've come this far with us, something must be working for you. Stay with us just a little longer, and we'll prove you can keep your weight loss on a steady and successful course. We'll also show you how to make the process even more enjoyable—not just the process of losing weight, but the process of *growth.* Some of your greatest rewards and pleasures will come from acquiring new knowledge, developing new self-management skills, and achieving new levels of fitness. We'll show you how to accomplish these goals at the same time you are reaching your ultimate weight-loss goal.

Why Change the Program?

The Continuity Phase of our program is based on exactly the same scientific principles as the 28-day Conditioning Phase you have just completed, and it relies on the same key behaviors for its success: reducing the fat in your diet, increasing the activity in your day, and changing your eating behaviors. But this phase differs significantly from the Conditioning Phase in several ways and for several reasons.

Your Body's Metabolic Changes

The primary reason for changing our program at this time is to adjust for the metabolic changes that are occurring in your body. As you lose weight, your body's weight regulator will start to "gear down" your metabolism to make up for your lighter weight and your lower caloric intake. This will cause you to burn slightly fewer calories each day. This is nature's way of trying to keep your weight at a constant level—in this case, too high a level. (See page 15 for a complete explanation of what occurs.)

This slowing of your metabolism doesn't mean that you'll stop losing weight, but it will decrease the speed at which you continue to lose it. Once you reach this stage, your weight loss—though slower than before—will tend to become a bit more steady and predictable.

When the rate of weight loss begins to slow, some people start doing dangerous things to speed it up again. They cut back drastically on their caloric intake (some even fast), which causes their body to destroy lean muscle tissue. Or they dramatically increase their exercise intensity and duration, which increases their risk of exhaustion and injury. The Continuity Phase of our program is designed to discourage you from doing those things, and to take your ongoing weight loss from body fat rather than muscle tissue.

Resetting Goals to Realistic Levels

When weight loss slows, many people—especially those who have a lot of weight to lose—become discouraged and abandon their program completely. All too often, these are people who have actually been quite successful at losing weight, but just don't recognize or appreciate their success. They lose a pound a week, week after week, and still quit because the weight is coming off more slowly than they had hoped for. Instead of enjoying their steady, small successes, they become discouraged and fall back on their old, unhealthy patterns of behavior. The Continuity Phase will help you avoid that mistake, because slow and consistent weight loss is the primary goal of the program.

To avoid the frustration that derails so many people at this point in their weight-loss efforts, it is important to set new goals for yourself that take into account your body's metabolic slowing. That does not mean you need to give up your ultimate weight-loss goal (assuming it was a reasonable one to begin with). But you must be willing to accept a realistic timetable for reaching that goal (for most people, that means a slower schedule). Using the Progress Charts in this chapter, you will be able to establish a definite schedule of weight loss for the weeks and months ahead. This will enable you to project the actual date when you will reach your final weight goal.

From Weight Loss to Fitness

Yet another reason to change our program now—perhaps the most important—is the need to expand the focus of your goals beyond weight loss to fitness. That may sound strange (it's likely you bought this book only because you wanted to lose weight), so let me explain the change in emphasis. When people become preoccupied with their weight alone, they lose sight of the other important benefits they are achieving as the excess pounds come off. Their energy levels increase, their muscle tone improves, their blood pressure and cholesterol levels drop, their clothes fit better—but they get no satisfaction from these results. In fact, some are so focused on their weight, they don't even notice the other good things that are happening.

This situation is especially troubling when it makes people who are actually successful in their weight-loss efforts *feel* as though they have failed. These people want to lose 50 pounds, but consider themselves failures if they lose only 30. Or they want to lose 15 pounds *quickly*, and get totally discouraged if it comes off slowly. As a consequence, they give up completely, and gain back not only the weight they've lost, but ten more pounds on top of it. Does that sound like anyone you know?

The Continuity Phase you are about to begin will help you avoid those mistakes by getting you to focus not only on your weight, but on other related issues that are at least as important—if not more so: your fitness level, your confidence level, your sense of control, and your comfort level. As you expand your focus to include other important outcomes, you will begin to feel more in control of your life, more confident about your abilities, and more comfortable with yourself—no matter what your weight.

Taking Responsibility for Your Own Results

During the 28-day Conditioning Phase of our program, you were given detailed assignments to follow every day. We did this to prove to you that small changes made over long periods of time would not only cause you to lose weight, but also improve your fitness level.

A rigid schedule like the one in our Conditioning Phase is certainly easy to follow and leaves no room for guesswork. But it also leaves little room for individual responsibility, which is so important for long-term success with weight control. So now it's time for you to take more responsibility.

To help you (or force you) to become more involved during the Continuity Phase, we'll switch from daily, rigid assignments to a weekly format with some suggested assignments. But there's room for flexibility: After 28 days on our program, you should be completely familiar with the scientific principles on which it is based, and you should know which specific activities work best for you.

Thus, feel free to take the assignments you'll find in this chapter, and adapt and fine-tune them so they fit into your own lifestyle, creating a more personalized program.

Think of the Continuity Phase as a training ground for independence. Unlike many weight-loss programs, which profit by keeping you dependent on their classes or packaged foods, our goal is to get you "on your own" as quickly as possible. The sooner you are able to create your own plan and structure for weight loss, the better. Let's get started on that goal now.

Getting Started

The first step in the Continuity Phase is to refocus your weight-loss goals, switching from the final weight you are trying to reach to a series of realistic intermediate weekly goals. Establishing these weekly goals is, in my opinion, one of the most essential steps you can take now. It forces you to be realistic about how long it will take you to reach your final goal. And being realistic now about the amount of time it takes to lose weight will keep you from getting discouraged and quitting later on. Being realistic about this issue now makes it possible to celebrate your progress in the coming weeks and months, instead of bemoaning the rate at which you are losing weight.

Just as important, setting weekly goals gives your Continuity Phase a solid structure you can use for monitoring your progress, and it makes your goals feel more achievable. Instead of focusing on distant and difficult goals, like losing 30 or 50 or even 100 pounds in a year, you can concentrate on achievable goals, like losing one pound in a week. If you do that every week for enough weeks, you'll be four pounds lighter in a month and you could be 52 pounds lighter in a year.

So what should your weekly goal be? And how can you even establish a weekly goal when you don't know how fast your remaining weight is going to come off? My advice is to make a conservative assumption, and be prepared to correct it later if you need to do so. At this point, simply assume that you will lose one pound per week until you reach your goal. With that assumption, you can now predict how much you will weigh next week and the week after and the week after that. In fact, by extending this assumption as far as you need to, you can now predict the exact week when you will reach your final goal.

How can you be sure you'll lose one pound a week? To be perfectly truthful, you can't. On the plan I'm about to lay out for you, the average person *will* lose about a pound per week, but some will lose more (especially people who are very heavy or very active or very careful about their fat intake) and some will lose less (people who are small, but heavy for their size, and people who are less active and less careful about their fat intake). Within a few weeks, you will find out which of the three groups you belong to.

If it does turn out that you lose exactly one pound per week, you should feel lucky. Don't make the mistake of trying to speed things up. What if you're losing *more* than a pound per week? Feel very lucky, but consider the possibility that you ought to slow down (I'll bet no weight-loss program ever told you to do that before). And what if you are losing less than a pound a week? Feel good. Feel successful. And, particularly if you are not a large person, feel *smart* for losing weight at a safe rate.

Now it's time to project what your weight will be in the coming weeks and months, to predict the week in which you will reach your final weight goal, and to become familiar with the charts you will use in the weeks ahead. Once you have done that, proceed to page 268 to begin the first week of your Continuity Phase.

Progress Charts

To monitor the Continuity Phase of your weight-loss program, you'll use one or more of the eight Progress Charts on the following pages. Step by step, chart by chart, here is how to use this system to keep track of your own progress:

Step 1: Along the left-hand edge of each graph, weight levels are listed in descending order—beginning at 300 pounds in the first graph, and continuing from one graph to the next, until it reaches 100 pounds in the last one. Turn to the chart on which you find your own weight listed in the left-hand column. From this point on, we'll refer to this chart as Progress Chart 1.

PROGRESS CHART I

Step 2: Enter today's date in the first date box in the top row of the chart.

Step 3: In the adjacent date boxes that run across the top of the chart, fill in the dates at weekly intervals from today's date. (Thus, if January 1 were the initial date you've entered, the next one would be January 8, followed by January 15, and so on.)

Step 4: In the left-hand column, find your current weight. Mark a black circle in the box where today's date and your current weight intersect.

Step 5: One week from today—and then in each subsequent week thereafter—enter a black circle indicating your weight on that date. Be sure to weigh yourself at the same time of day each week (preferably first thing in the morning).

Step 6: Connect these black circles with a diagonal line, which will clearly show the direction of your progress.

Step 7: When you have reached the last date on the top of the chart—or if your weight has declined to the bottom row on the grid—then move to the next chart (Progress Chart 2) if you still have more weight to lose. (Or if you finished the 25-week period in the middle of Chart 1, continue to monitor your progress by writing in new dates and circles in a different color.)

PROGRESS CHART 2

Step 8: Write a new set of dates at the top of this chart. The first date should be one week after the last date on Progress Chart 1, and subsequent dates should be one week apart.

Step 9: On the first date of Progress Chart 2, weigh yourself, and find this weight in the left-hand column. Mark a black circle in the square where the date and your weight intersect.

Step 10: On each subsequent date on this chart, make a black circle indicating your weight on that date. Again, be sure to weigh yourself at the same time of day each week (first thing in the morning, if possible).

Step 11: Connect the black circles with a diagonal line, which will show the direction of your progress.

Step 12: When you have reached the last date on the top of the chart—or if your weight has declined to the bottom row on the grid—then move to the next chart if you still have more weight to lose.

PROGRESS CHART 3 AND BEYOND

Step 13: Write a new set of dates at the top of this chart, as you did in the previous one.

Step 14+: Continue the process of weighing and charting, moving from week to week and from chart to chart until you reach your weight-loss goal.

PROGRESS CHART

PROGRESS CHART

Wt	Week 1	2	3	4	5	6	7	8	9	10	11	12	13	14	15	16	17	18	19	20	21	22	23	24	25	Wt
300																										300
299																										299
298																										298
297																										297
296																										296
295																										295
294																										294
293																										293
292																										292
291																										291
290																										290
289																										289
288																										288
287																										287
286																										286
285																										285
284																										284
283																										283
282																										282
281																										281
280																										280
279																										279
278																										278
277																										277
276																										276
275																										275

Date

PROGRESS CHART

PROGRESS CHART

PROGRESS CHART

Date																											
Wt	1	2	3	4	5	6	7	8	9	10	11	12	13	14	15	16	17	18	19	20	21	22	23	24	25		Wt
275																											275
274																											274
273																											273
272																											272
271																											271
270																											270
269																											269
268																											268
267																											267
266																											266
265																											265
264																											264
263																											263
262																											262
261																											261
260																											260
259																											259
258																											258
257																											257
256																											256
255																											255
254																											254
253																											253
252																											252
251																											251
250																											250
Week	1	2	3	4	5	6	7	8	9	10	11	12	13	14	15	16	17	18	19	20	21	22	23	24	25		Week

PROGRESS CHART

PROGRESS CHART

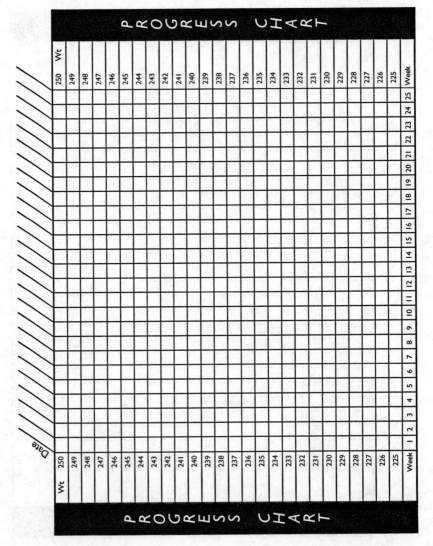

PROGRESS CHART

PROGRESS CHART

Wt	1	2	3	4	5	6	7	8	9	10	11	12	13	14	15	16	17	18	19	20	21	22	23	24	25	Wt
225																										225
224																										224
223																										223
222																										222
221																										221
220																										220
219																										219
218																										218
217																										217
216																										216
215																										215
214																										214
213																										213
212																										212
211																										211
210																										210
209																										209
208																										208
207																										207
206																										206
205																										205
204																										204
203																										203
202																										202
201																										201
200																										200
Week	1	2	3	4	5	6	7	8	9	10	11	12	13	14	15	16	17	18	19	20	21	22	23	24	25	Week

Date

PROGRESS CHART

PROGRESS CHART

P R O G R E S S   C H A R T

Date																									Wt
																									200
																									199
																									198
																									197
																									196
																									195
																									194
																									193
																									192
																									191
																									190
																									189
																									188
																									187
																									186
																									185
																									184
																									183
																									182
																									181
																									180
																									179
																									178
																									177
																									176
																									175
Week	1	2	3	4	5	6	7	8	9	10	11	12	13	14	15	16	17	18	19	20	21	22	23	24	25

P R O G R E S S   C H A R T

PROGRESS CHART

PROGRESS CHART

Date

Wt	Week	1	2	3	4	5	6	7	8	9	10	11	12	13	14	15	16	17	18	19	20	21	22	23	24	25	Week	Wt
175																												175
174																												174
173																												173
172																												172
171																												171
170																												170
169																												169
168																												168
167																												167
166																												166
165																												165
164																												164
163																												163
162																												162
161																												161
160																												160
159																												159
158																												158
157																												157
156																												156
155																												155
154																												154
153																												153
152																												152
151																												151
150																												150

PROGRESS CHART

PROGRESS CHART

PROGRESS CHART

Wt	1	2	3	4	5	6	7	8	9	10	11	12	13	14	15	16	17	18	19	20	21	22	23	24	25	Wt
150																										150
149																										149
148																										148
147																										147
146																										146
145																										145
144																										144
143																										143
142																										142
141																										141
140																										140
139																										139
138																										138
137																										137
136																										136
135																										135
134																										134
133																										133
132																										132
131																										131
130																										130
129																										129
128																										128
127																										127
126																										126
125																										125
Week	1	2	3	4	5	6	7	8	9	10	11	12	13	14	15	16	17	18	19	20	21	22	23	24	25	Week

Date

PROGRESS CHART

PROGRESS CHART

Wt	1	2	3	4	5	6	7	8	9	10	11	12	13	14	15	16	17	18	19	20	21	22	23	24	25	Wt
125																										125
124																										124
123																										123
122																										122
121																										121
120																										120
119																										119
118																										118
117																										117
116																										116
115																										115
114																										114
113																										113
112																										112
111																										111
110																										110
109																										109
108																										108
107																										107
106																										106
105																										105
104																										104
103																										103
102																										102
101																										101
100																										100
Week	1	2	3	4	5	6	7	8	9	10	11	12	13	14	15	16	17	18	19	20	21	22	23	24	25	Week

Date

PROGRESS CHART

A Hypothetical Case

To help you better understand how these charts should be utilized, let's look at how an individual named Jane used them. When she began the Continuity Phase of this program, she weighed 165 pounds. Her goal weight was 135—a loss of a pound a week for the next 30 weeks.

Step 1: Jane turned to the chart on which she found 165 pounds listed in the left-hand margin. This became her Progress Chart 1.

JANE'S PROGRESS CHART I

Step 2: Jane entered the present date in the first column across the top of the chart. In this case, Jane wrote February 1.

Step 3: In the adjacent columns, Jane filled in the subsequent dates at weekly intervals, starting with February 8, February 15, February 22, and so on.

Step 4: In the vertical column under February 1, Jane found her present weight (165 pounds), and made a black circle in the square where the date and her weight intersected.

Step 5: A week later, on February 8, Jane got on the scale in the morning shortly after awakening. Her weight was 164 pounds, so she made a black circle where her weight and the date intersected.

Step 6: In subsequent weeks—on February 15, 22, and so on— Jane weighed herself in the morning, and noted her weight with black circles on the grid. She continued to lose weight at a pace of one pound per week.

Step 7: Jane connected the black circles with a diagonal line, which provided a clear visual picture of her downward direction of steady weight loss.

Step 8: On week 16, Jane's weight had reached 150 pounds—the bottom row on the grid of Progress Chart 1. Since she still had more weight to lose, she moved to the next chart.

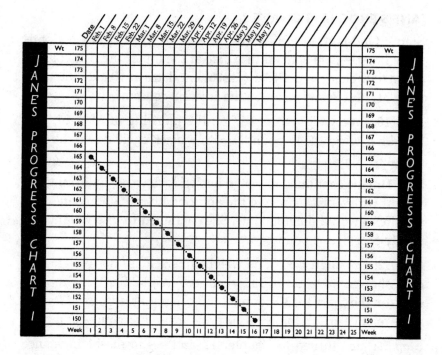

JANE'S PROGRESS CHART 2

Step 9: On May 24—which was the start of week 17 of her Continuity Phase—Jane entered that date at the top of the first column of the new chart, and wrote subsequent dates at weekly intervals (May 31, June 7, and so on) in the adjacent columns.

Step 10: Jane weighed herself on the morning of May 24, and noted her weight (149 pounds) with a black circle down the first column of the chart.

Step 11: Jane continued to weigh herself each week, indicating her weight with a black circle in the appropriate box, and connecting the circles with a diagonal line. She continued to lose weight at a steady pace of one pound a week.

Step 12: On August 30, Jane weighed herself. To her delight, the scale showed a weight of 135—her goal weight! She drew a black circle on the chart at 135 pounds, and congratulated herself for her perseverance in sticking with the program and reaching her target.

Step 13: Jane turned to Chapter 12, and began the Maintenance Phase of this book.

JANE'S PROGRESS CHART 2

Date: May 24, May 31, June 7, June 14, June 21, June 28, July 5, July 12, July 19, July 26, Aug. 2, Aug. 9, Aug. 16, Aug. 23, Aug. 30

| Wt | 150 | 149 | 148 | 147 | 146 | 145 | 144 | 143 | 142 | 141 | 140 | 139 | 138 | 137 | 136 | 135 | 134 | 133 | 132 | 131 | 130 | 129 | 128 | 127 | 126 | 125 |

| Week | 1 | 2 | 3 | 4 | 5 | 6 | 7 | 8 | 9 | 10 | 11 | 12 | 13 | 14 | 15 | 16 | 17 | 18 | 19 | 20 | 21 | 22 | 23 | 24 | 25 |

Case Studies

Some people do not lose at this steady rate of a pound a week. Instead, their weight declines more slowly or more rapidly than predicted, or their weight fluctuates up and down. Here is a look at some deviations from the norm, and what course of correction can be taken:

PROGRESS CHART A:
WEIGHT LOSS SLOWER THAN PREDICTED BUT STEADY

This chart shows a loss of eight pounds in 24 weeks. That is less weight than the pound-per-week originally predicted, but the slope of the weight-loss line shows that the weight is coming off quite steadily. There could be several explanations for this outcome: (1) the suggested assignments (or assignments the individual created herself) are only being partially followed—especially the reduction of dietary fat; (2) this could be the chart of a small person or an older person (these people tend to lose weight more slowly); (3) the person could be very close to the final goal weight (the weight regulating system will resist further weight loss even more vigorously). In the first case, greater restriction of fat might be useful. In the last two cases, further dietary restriction could be harmful; patience is called for.

PROGRESS CHART A

Date

Wt	1	2	3	4	5	6	7	8	9	10	11	12	13	14	15	16	17	18	19	20	21	22	23	24	25
150																									
149																									
148																									
147																									
146																									
145	●																								
144		●	●		●																				
143				●	●		●																		
142								●	●	●		●													
141											●		●												
140														●	●	●			●	●					
139																	●	●			●				
138																						●	●		
137																								●	
136																									
135																									
134																									
133																									
132																									
131																									
130																									
129																									
128																									
127																									
126																									
125																									
Week	1	2	3	4	5	6	7	8	9	10	11	12	13	14	15	16	17	18	19	20	21	22	23	24	25

PROGRESS CHART B:
WEIGHT LOSS SLOWER THAN PREDICTED AND UNSTEADY

This chart also shows a loss of eight pounds in 25 weeks, but the slope of the weight-loss line is very erratic. This person is rapidly losing and gaining weight in fits and spurts, with the losses only slightly ahead of the gains. This pattern suggests a person who is alternating excessive caloric restriction with intermittent over-indulgence. This pattern is dangerous because of the risk that lean muscle tissue is being destroyed during the periods of rapid weight loss, while additional fat tissue is being stored in the body during the periods of weight gain.

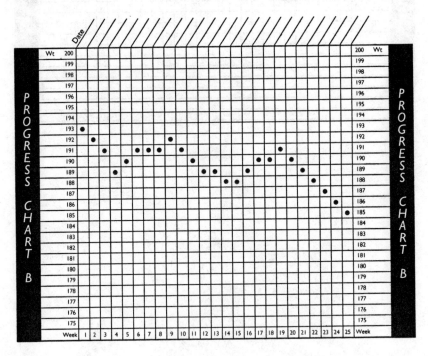

PROGRESS CHART C:
WEIGHT LOSS FASTER THAN PREDICTED

This chart shows a loss of 24 pounds in 16 weeks, significantly more than originally predicted. Note that the weight loss is taking place at a very steady pace. This rate of weight loss would be considered reasonable in a person who was extremely heavy (for example, more than 150 pounds overweight). However, it would be considered too rapid—and unsafe—in a woman who was five feet tall and started out weighing 135 pounds, for example. Weight loss of this magnitude may be a sign of excessive caloric restriction, which can produce muscle destruction and nutritional deficiency.

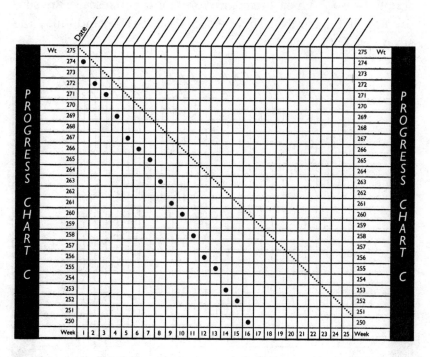

PROGRESS CHART D:
WEIGHT LOSS AS PREDICTED, BUT ERRATIC

This chart shows a person whose weight, at first glance, appears to be going up and down, but who is actually steadily losing weight at the rate of about one pound per week. The pattern seen on this chart can be explained in several ways: (1) The individual could be weighing herself on different days of the week or at different times of the day (people tend to weigh more at night than in the morning; they may weigh more after weekends than after weekdays); (2) varying levels of salt intake could be producing occasional episodes of fluid retention; (3) the differences could simply be due to measurement errors (most home scales are simply not that accurate). This person should relax and enjoy the steady weight loss.

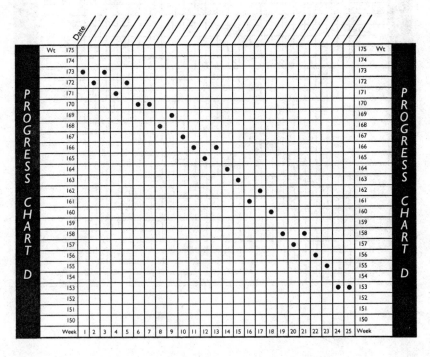

Implementing the Continuity Phase

Until you have reached your goal weight, follow this Continuity Phase, not only by filling in the Progress Charts to keep track of your weight loss, but by using the tear-out Self-Monitoring charts in the book to help you detect any problem areas that arise.

In the following pages, you'll find the information and assignments to carry you through the next ten weeks. (If you still haven't reached your goal after those ten weeks, repeat the basic assignments in Week 10 until you do.) Each week, in addition to the assignments, you'll find a guiding success principle that will help you in your efforts to lose all the weight you want to lose. Use these strategies throughout the Continuity Phase. Also, throughout the chapter, you'll read about the accomplishments of our original TODAY show participants, and how they are using these ten principles in their own weight-loss efforts.

WEEK I

Success Principle #1

FOLLOWING A CONCRETE PLAN

Adhering to a definite plan is one of the most important things you can do to increase your chance of losing weight and keeping it off. A plan defines what you must do to reach your goal, eliminating some of the guesswork. A plan that is too rigid, however, can be self-defeating, because it becomes too difficult to follow. A rigid plan also tends to make you a more passive participant in the weight-loss process, and leaves you less prepared to deal with problems when you go off the program. Long-term success in losing and keeping weight off depends on your learning how to make healthy choices for yourself.

The plan you should be following in the Continuity Phase contains two elements to guide you: a set of general principles in four key areas (decreasing fat, increasing activity, changing eating behaviors, and monitoring), and a daily set of assignments in each area. In the long run, the general principles will enable you to create your own plan for long-term weight maintenance, so that you can keep off the weight that you are continuing to lose.

The Importance of Structure: Anne Langley

Anne Langley's recent weight-loss experience illustrates the importance of maintaining a structured program until you reach your ultimate weight-loss goal. She enjoyed early success during the first 28 days of our plan, while we were providing her with precise daily assignments to follow, and she kept it up during the first few weeks thereafter, maintaining a 15-pound weight loss right up to the three-month mark. But without following a formal program after that, Anne eventually began running into problems.

"I'm the type of person who needs structure," she said. "And the program provided that structure for me. But after the first 28 days, even though I was able to keep going for a while, I soon began having lapses. I no longer felt accountable, and I went through several periods of stops and starts."

Anne, a registered nurse, has been overweight—and dieting—since her teenage years. But when she joined our volunteer weight-control group, she was optimistic about her chances of success.

Almost immediately, Anne began losing weight, and exercise seemed to be a key. For years, she had been limiting the fat in her diet, but she had never really been physically active. Our daily assignments during the first 28 days prompted her to begin a walking program, which soon progressed to jogging. "I enjoyed exercising so much, and it gave me so much extra energy," she said. "It also made me feel in control and kept me motivated. I had always heard that for exercise to have any benefit, you had to push yourself to the point of exhaustion. It was such a relief to find out that the intensity wasn't that important; it was the distance and the frequency that mattered."

Once our formal 28-day program was over, however, and without a Continuity Phase in place, Anne's difficulties surfaced. Exercise was the first thing to go, because there were no longer any mandatory distances to cover. Once the discipline of regular exercise was lost, everything else seemed to drift away, too. "When I didn't exercise, I no longer felt I even had a program," she said. Six months after she first joined us in the weight-loss plan, Anne had gained back seven of the 15 pounds she had lost. Eventually, all of the weight she had lost came back—and a few pounds more.

When Anne's weight was at its high point, we discussed the difficulties she was having, and I convinced her to begin walking again, even just very short distances in the first few days, and to consider herself back on the program. The last time we talked, she was exercising regularly. Seven mornings a week, between 6:00 and 7:00, she puts on her workout clothes and walks for 45 to 90 minutes. "I enjoy the quiet of the morning, and I'm walking in all kinds of weather, even snow and ice." She is also participating in an aerobics class twice a week.

Anne's return to a structured exercise program has gotten her back on track with every other aspect of her weight-loss plan. Even when she slips a little elsewhere, the exercise helps her compensate for it. "Now, if I occasionally eat something that I consider inappropriate, I feel that the exercise makes up for it," said Anne. "It keeps everything in check."

The weight is coming off again, with a seven-pound loss in the weeks just before this was written. Anne credits her structured exercise program, which seems to be working even when she oversleeps occasionally and skips a session. "When that happens, I really feel as though I've missed something essential," she said. "Exercise has become very important in my life again. I'm glad to be back in the swing of things."

Week 1

Assignment

1. Decrease fat in your diet so it accounts for less than 20 percent of your total calories for the day. To accomplish this, increase your intake of foods that have 10 percent or less of their calories from fat, and cut back significantly on foods with 30 percent or more of their calories from fat.

2. Cover at least three miles each day (walking or running at any pace, continuously or in smaller segments), or substitute any equivalent activity.

3. Walk up at least four flights of stairs.

4. Eat your meals using the pacing system, pausing 30 seconds between each bite.

5. Eat at least three meals a day.

6. Using the Self-Monitoring charts, score yourself at the end of each day for goals accomplished.

7. To comply with this week's Success Principle, take time now to create a concrete written plan for dealing with any areas of our program that are causing problems for you. Reflect on the thoughts below to help you organize your plan.

   - Problems that got in my way
   - Strategies to overcome problems
   - Triggers to be aware of
   - Rewards: What did I do for myself?
   - What am I planning to do for myself?

WEEK 2

Success Principle #2

BEING PATIENT AND ACCEPTING SLOW PROGRESS

Most overweight people want to lose their excess weight rapidly. Unfortunately, rapid weight loss—even under medical supervision—is more hazardous than gradual loss. People who lose weight very quickly are much more prone to medical complications, including gallstones, dehydration, vitamin and mineral depletion, and abnormal heart rhythms.

People whose weight declines very rapidly are also more likely to regain the weight they have lost. In part, that's because some weight-loss plans (usually not the medically supervised ones) accomplish their dramatic losses not just by eliminating body fat, but by destroying lean muscle tissue as well. Since muscle tissue contains so much more water than fatty tissue, weight drops rapidly. However, as soon as you start eating normally again and replacing the muscle tissue that was lost, the weight returns just as quickly as it disappeared.

Weight-loss plans that promise dramatic, rapid results usually involve extremely low-calorie diets or fasting. These plans often ignore the psychological, emotional, and behavioral issues that influence your weight regulator. As long as you follow the extreme diet, the weight comes off. But as soon as you return to your usual diet, the pounds will creep back on again if you are unprepared to deal with the other issues that influence your weight. Slowly but surely, your weight regulator will drag your weight back up to the set point it has chosen for you.

The road to long-term weight-loss success is not measured in pounds, but in fractions of ounces; not in days or weeks, but in years and decades. Skipping just a single bite of food at each meal can have a dramatic effect. If you left one 25-calorie bite of food on your plate at every meal, by the end of a year you would lose eight pounds. The effect of regular low-intensity exercise is just as significant: A mile a day for a year is worth ten pounds on the scale.

An old saying applies here: Count the pennies, and the dollars will take care of themselves. Making these small changes a regular part of your daily routine will produce very substantial weight loss over time. The effects are even more impressive when you combine the different activities that form the core of our program.

A few more examples show how modest adjustments in your food choices and physical activity can add up to significant weight loss over the long run.

- Substitute a three-ounce baked potato for three ounces of French fries, three times a week, and you could lose eight and a half pounds a year.

- Drink 3 cups of skim milk a day instead of 3 cups of whole milk, and you could lose 20 pounds a year.

- Substitute three ounces of halibut for three ounces of prime rib of beef, once a week, and you could lose three and a half pounds a year.

- Instead of three ounces of potato chips once a week, have 3 cups of air-popped popcorn, and you could lose nearly six pounds a year.

Enjoying Gradual Weight Loss: Patti Garrett

When Patti Garrett joined our weight-loss program, she told me about the diets she had tried in the past, all of which had left her feeling even worse about herself than before she had started them. "I tried commercial weight-loss programs, and when I didn't lose weight fast enough, they made me feel like a failure; and when I gained weight, they made me feel even worse," said Patti. When we asked her, "How would you feel if you lost weight, but it was just one or two pounds?" she responded, "I'd feel like a failure."

Patti was unwilling to accept anything but perfection, and saw no value in achieving anything short of her ultimate goal. Perhaps more than anything, we helped her recognize and appreciate even the small successes she had. Over the weeks, she learned to be more patient, and to accept even slow progress as a success. We kept telling her that every intermediate step on the way to her goal was meaningful, and she finally began to see it that way.

In fact, on our plan, Patti lost 18 pounds in the first three months. She regained three of them by the six-month reunion—something she would have seen as a failure in the past. With her new outlook, she focused instead with pride on the 15 pounds she had kept off.

"The key for me was the support I got," she said. "Dr. Ulene's staff didn't make me feel bad when things weren't going perfectly. Rather than saying something like, 'What did you do wrong this time?' they reminded me, 'Start again tomorrow; next week is going to be a better week.' They kept my attitude very positive and helped me put everything in perspective, including enjoying the successes I was having, and being patient rather than insisting on losing the weight almost overnight."

We told Patti that she had a choice—she could blame herself for any setbacks, and call herself a failure; or she could focus on what she had accomplished to that point. She got her first real test when she developed asthma and bronchitis—conditions that made it much harder for her to exercise. Up to that time, she had been participating in a step aerobics class at the George Washington University Obesity Management Program, and she walked outdoors as well. But her breathing problems became worse when she exercised vigorously, and her doctor advised her to avoid walking in the hot, humid summer weather. For three months, she stopped exercising altogether, and the medication she was taking—prednisone—actually tended to push her weight upward.

In the past, Patti would have considered this turn of events a sign of failure, and she would have abandoned all of her weight-loss efforts. But today, she continues to focus instead on the successes she has had to date. She now views the asthma as a temporary obstacle, and has concentrated her attention on low-fat eating to help her maintain about a 15-pound weight loss. "I'm still feeling strong, and I'm hopeful that once my physical condition improves and I can work out again, I'm going to continue to lose more." Meanwhile, she's proud of being able to keep her weight just where it is.

Week 2

Assignment

1. Decrease fat in your diet so it accounts for less than 20 percent of your total calories for the day. To accomplish this, increase your intake of foods that have 10 percent or less of their calories from fat, and cut back significantly on foods with 30 percent or more of their calories from fat.

2. Cover at least three miles each day (walking or running at any pace, continuously or in smaller segments), or substituting any equivalent activity.

3. Walk up at least four flights of stairs.

4. Eat your meals using the pacing system, pausing 30 seconds between each bite.

5. Eat at least three meals a day.

6. Using the Self-Monitoring charts, score yourself at the end of each day for goals accomplished.

7. To reinforce this week's Success Principle, calculate how much you will weigh on the dates listed below, assuming that you will lose weight at the rate of one pound per week. Enter your projected weights in the spaces below:

President's Day	_____	Christmas Day	_____
Memorial Day	_____	New Year's Day	_____
Labor Day	_____	Your Birthday	_____
Thanksgiving Day	_____	My Birthday (July 13)	_____

Copy these dates and weights down on a card or sheet of paper and post it or place it where you can conveniently refer to it. This list of dates and weights will serve as a reminder that you will ultimately reach your goal if you just stay with the program.

WEEK 3

Success Principle #3

PAYING ACTIVE ATTENTION TO EATING

It is surprising how little attention most of us pay to the act of eating. If asked, we could probably describe most of the meals we ate during the day, and we would probably remember how much food we consumed. But many of us would have difficulty describing how each bite tasted, or what we were thinking at the time we took each bite.

In some respects, eating is much like driving a car. We drive from place to place almost automatically, stopping without thinking when signals turn red, and braking reflexively whenever traffic slows. When we get to our destination, few of us can produce any details about how we got there or what we passed along the way.

Though certainly conscious of eating, we are usually not actively attentive to the process. We let our minds drift or become preoccupied with other issues. We miss much of the sensory pleasure that food has to offer. We also lose track of how much food we are eating. As a result, we eat more than we really need or want.

An essential element of the Continuity Phase is the same pacing program used in the first 28 days, which is designed to increase your attention to eating. This pacing program helps you slow your eating speed, so you have time to pay attention to the process of eating. It also helps you deliberately focus attention on the sensory qualities of your food (its appearance, taste, aroma, and consistency).

For many people, using the pacing program continues to be one of the most difficult components of this plan—even though it should be one of the easiest. If you had been used to eating quickly, the amount of time you have been asked to spend between bites might have seemed interminable. You may have been used to eating while reading or watching television; the pacing program makes either activity impossible. If you are ravenously hungry when you sit down to eat, the temptation will still be great to consume large quantities of food immediately. If other rapid eaters are with you at the table, they may complain about your "slowness."

Whatever happens to make you consider abandoning the pacing program, I urge you not to do so. After 28 days, you should be conditioning yourself to accept the new pace, and it should begin to feel natural. If you are eating too rapidly now, remember that you have spent a lifetime practicing that pace. Give yourself time to learn what a new pace can feel like.

Changing Eating Behaviors: Ed Caffery

Ed Caffery was enthusiastic about this weight-loss program from day one. But even he has been surprised by just how much long-term success he has enjoyed. Three months after joining the TODAY show group, Ed had lost 38 pounds—but that was only the beginning. At the six-month point, he was down 50 pounds, and he has continued to lose about one pound a month since then.

There are many reasons for Ed's success, but his active attention to his eating behavior is one of the most important, including his focus on how fast he eats. "I eat a lot slower now than I once did, especially when I'm eating with my daughter, who also is participating in the program," he said. "It's difficult to do sometimes, yet by eating only half as fast as I did before, I'm paying attention to everything I eat, and I'm not allowing myself to be distracted by reading the newspaper while eating."

For the first few weeks of the program, Ed affixed the word "pacing" to the dashboard of his car as a reminder. "It's a great idea to pace yourself in everything in life, not just eating," he said. "And by spending even a small amount of time thinking about the pacing system, it helps bring all the rest of the weight-loss program into focus."

As part of Ed's active attention to eating, he has developed a taste for lower-fat foods that, at one time, he might have never considered palatable. "I liked plain old bologna, which can run about 100 calories per slice, with a fat content of 80 percent," he recalled.

Then he made the switch to non-fat bologna, which has just 20 calories a slice. Sure, it doesn't taste exactly the same, he says, but he's gotten used to it, and he feels good about making wiser, healthier choices.

Ed has also become an avid exerciser. "I usually awaken at 5:30, and before I have a cup of coffee or a conversation with my wife, or before opening the morning paper to see how the Orioles are doing, I get on my exercise bike for 30 minutes or more. Yes, there are days when I don't feel like exercising, but I'll force myself to do at least ten minutes, which often extends to 30. Or I might get my exercise for the day in three separate ten-minute sessions."

This isn't the first time Ed has tried to lose weight. He says that he's taken off 80 pounds on at least three different occasions, and has lost 20 pounds about ten other times. But until now, he has never been able to keep it off for an extended period. "I always lost it in a hurry, and then put it back on in a hurry," he said.

Now that Ed appreciates the importance of pacing and the other components of this program, he is much happier with his continuing loss of just one pound per month. "A pound a month may not sound like enormous progress," he said. "But the real progress for me is that I haven't put a pound a month—or five pounds a month—back on! And I'm continuing to lose!"

Ed describes this program as "not only possible but also painless." In recent years, he had been hospitalized three times for problems with asthma, but his condition is much better, and his doctor believes the weight loss has helped.

Ed ended a recent letter to me with the following line: "You just may have saved my life and certainly made it a lot better life."

Week 3

Assignment

1. Decrease fat in your diet so it accounts for less than 20 percent of your total calories for the day. To accomplish this, increase your intake of foods that have 10 percent or less of their calories from fat, and cut back significantly on foods with 30 percent or more of their calories from fat.

2. Cover at least three miles each day (walking or running at any pace, continuously or in smaller segments), or substitute any equivalent activity.

3. Walk up at least four flights of stairs.

4. Eat your meals using the pacing system, pausing 30 seconds between each bite.

5. Eat at least three meals a day.

6. Using the Self-Monitoring charts, score yourself at the end of each day for goals accomplished.

7. To see how you are doing with this week's Success Principle, time yourself during at least one meal each day to determine the interval between your bites. Measure the duration of your meal in minutes and keep an accurate count of the number of bites you take. Divide the number of minutes by the number of bites to calculate the interval between bites (for example: if you took 20 bites in ten minutes, you would divide ten by 20; the interval is 30 seconds per bite). If your interval is less than 30 seconds per bite, work on a strategy for slowing down. If necessary, use a watch or clock with a second hand to time each bite you take.

WEEK 4

Success Principle #4

RECOVERING QUICKLY WHEN YOU LAPSE

No matter how clear your weight-loss plan or how strong your resolve, chances are you'll slip off the Continuity Phase once in a while. Everyone does. The reasons for lapses are many: pressures at work or home; tempting restaurant fare; parties, celebrations, holidays. The list of plan-busting opportunities goes on and on. As soon as you "take advantage" of those opportunities, the weight goes on, too. Before long, the small slip that put an extra pound or so on your frame can become a long slide that packs on more.

It's unrealistic to expect that you'll never slip, but you must not let a little lapse in behavior turn into a total relapse and abandonment of all your weight-loss efforts. Remember the lesson that successful people have taught us: Don't wait even one extra minute to begin your recovery. Put aside any disappointment, frustration, or anger you are feeling with yourself or the plan you are following. Swallow your pride (instead of more food), and get back on your plan immediately.

Treat each slip as a warning sign that something has gone awry. Analyze the events leading up to your lapse. Was it stress, over-work, exposure to high-fat foods at holiday parties? Did you overdo exercise to the point of pain, and then give up completely? The more you understand about the cause of your setback, the greater the likelihood that it won't happen again. Take time, also, to pre-pare a preventive plan you can use the next time you encounter the same circumstances.

Through it all, stay optimistic. A positive attitude is important for a quick recovery. The faster you refocus your attention on your accomplishments rather than your failures, the more rapidly you will reach and maintain your ultimate weight-loss goal. Set aside any need you have to be perfect—and accept the fact that you are human.

At the same time, recommit yourself to this program. Beginning with your next meal, choose low-fat foods once again. Resume your exercise program, restore your eating pace—return to the plan as though nothing had happened. The sooner you put yourself back on track after a lapse, the less impact the lapse will have.

Rebounding from Setbacks: Phyllis Mazer

Nearly everyone has lapses and setbacks, where they regain some (and sometimes all) of the weight they've lost. But Phyllis Mazer wasn't prepared for just how rapidly those pounds could return.

Phyllis had dropped 16 pounds on our program, losing it gradually and keeping it off for many months. "I learned so much about how to lose weight, and everything just seemed to fall into place," she said.

But unexpectedly, Phyllis developed an abscessed tooth, which caused swelling, tenderness, and extreme pain in her mouth and face. For weeks, she struggled with this dental problem, ultimately taking antibiotics for 40 days to clear up the stubborn infection.

During this lengthy ordeal, Phyllis became so distracted by the constant pain that she found it virtually impossible to exercise and pay attention to her diet. It was hard to find foods she could comfortably eat, and ice cream became one of the few foods that was tolerable and even soothing.

Six weeks after her dental problems began, and after a root canal procedure was ultimately performed, Phyllis was finally pain-free—but she had regained all of the 16 pounds she had lost, and even a little more. Still, she didn't let her disappointment overwhelm her. Instead, she immediately decided to start the recovery process.

"I had regained the weight, but I really wasn't upset about the poor food choices I had made," said Phyllis. "In the past, I might have cried about it. But I didn't have a sense of guilt this time. It was something that happened, and I just made the decision to get back on the program."

Phyllis used our pacing audiotapes to help her slow her eating speed, and she began concentrating on low-fat foods again. She started exercising seven days a week, 30 minutes a day, in her backyard pool. And she added some walking to her schedule as well.

About a week after Phyllis had climbed back on the road to recovery, she told us that the lapse was behind her and she had already lost two pounds. "This is one of the best programs I've been on," she said. "I have all the skills I need to lose weight, and I'm determined that the setback I had isn't going to keep me from enjoying long-term success."

Week 4

Assignment

1. Decrease fat in your diet so it accounts for less than 20 percent of your total calories for the day. To accomplish this, increase your intake of foods that have 10 percent or less of their calories from fat, and cut back significantly on foods with 30 percent or more of their calories from fat.

2. Cover at least three miles each day (walking or running at any pace, continuously or in smaller segments), or substitute any equivalent activity.

3. Walk up at least four flights of stairs.

4. Eat your meals using the pacing system, pausing 30 seconds between each bite.

5. Eat at least three meals a day.

6. Using the Self-Monitoring charts, score yourself at the end of each day for goals accomplished.

7. To prepare yourself for implementing this week's Success Principle, commit yourself to maintain an optimistic, positive attitude during any future lapses and sign the commitment form provided below.

Personal Commitment

If I deviate from my plan, I hereby commit myself to return to the plan within 24 hours. If I do return to the plan within that time frame, I promise to reward myself in the following way: Stay in bed late and read or watch TV; invite a friend to a movie; buy myself a new piece of clothing; _____.

(fill in your own reward suggestions)

_____

Your Signature

WEEK 5

Success Principle #5

EATING A LOW-FAT DIET

Of all the actions that can lead to long-term weight loss, reducing your dietary fat is not only the simplest but, from a medical point of view, one of the most important. Eating a low-fat diet will decrease your risk of high blood cholesterol, coronary heart disease, and colon cancer. It is also one of the most effective ways you can lose weight and keep it off.

In the first 28 days, you learned that high-fat foods deliver huge amounts of calories in very small portions. You can eat a considerably larger quantity of low-fat food while still losing weight. Furthermore, if on a given day your caloric intake does exceed your energy expenditure, you are much less likely to store the excess calories as fat if there is little fat in your diet.

Cutting the fat in your diet is an easy way to rebalance your weight-regulating system, compared to changing your exercise levels or eating behaviors. Switching from three glasses of whole milk to three glasses of nonfat has the same weight-loss effect as running one and a half miles, but it's a lot less work. And there are literally hundreds of ways to reduce the quantity of fat you're consuming without making any great sacrifices.

The other nice thing about cutting fat out of your diet is that it grows on you. It may be hard to believe how greasy whole milk will taste after you've been drinking only nonfat for a few months—or how much better fresh bread will taste without butter or margarine after you've eaten bread plain for a while.

During the 28-day program, I hope you made a habit of reducing your daily fat intake so it accounted for less than 20 percent of the calories you consumed. One way to continue to accomplish this goal is to count all of the calories you are consuming throughout the day, accounting separately for fat calories and those derived from protein and carbohydrates. Without question, this is the most precise way to calculate the percentage of calories that come from fat; unfortunately, it is also very laborious.

For those who cannot afford the time it takes to count every calorie, I still encourage you to use the much simpler, though less precise, system that uses the law of averages to help you reach the 20 percent goal. Here, again, is how it works.

- You will eliminate, or cut back drastically on, foods that derive more than 30 percent of their calories from fat.

- You will significantly increase your intake of foods that derive 10 percent or less of their calories from fat.

- You will eat the remaining foods (which derive 11 to 29 percent of their calories from fat) thoughtfully and carefully.

By following these three simple guidelines, your overall fat calorie intake should stay well below the 20 percent goal you are working toward. In our experience, some people have brought their actual fat consumption down to 10 percent levels using only these guidelines.

To assist you in determining which foods contain more than 30 percent or less than 10 percent of their calories in the form of fat, use the examples listed throughout this book. But you will obviously need considerably more information to make decisions about the wide variety of food choices that confront you. Much of this information is now available on the new nutrition labels of packaged foods. But you may have to do a little more research to determine the percentage of fat in other foods, such as meats, poultry, and fish, or in foods served in restaurants. I strongly recommend that you purchase a "counter" book that lists the fat content of foods, and use it at the end of each day to check the foods you chose at the market or in restaurants. Better yet, carry one of these books with you if you can, and check on fat content *before* selecting foods. Be sure to pick a book that lists not only the number of fat grams contained in foods, but also the percent of calories that come from fat. This information will save you from doing all the calculations yourself.

The extra effort you make to learn about the fat content of the foods you are eating will be well rewarded. You'll find that you lose excess pounds much more steadily, and you'll be much more likely to keep them off. In a short time, this part of your weight-loss plan will become literally effortless as you learn the amount of fat in various foods and no longer have to look these values up.

Every day, use the the Self-Monitoring charts to monitor your accomplishments in this critical area of the program. If you ate no foods containing more than 30 percent of calories from fat (or only very few of those foods, in very small portions), you will fill in the entire circle that represents your fat-reducing activities for the day on the chart. If you go off the plan entirely, you will leave the circle blank. If you fall somewhere in between, color in half the circle. Don't worry about precision. As in the first 28 days, your approximations will soon reveal how well you are doing in this area, and where your problems lie.

Choosing a Low-Fat Lifestyle: Art Dow

Unlike many people who have adopted our weight-control program, Art Dow was never a chronic dieter. On our program, Art dropped 11 pounds—a weight loss that might seem modest at first glance, but it had a significant effect upon his physical well-being. Art had high blood pressure, and just the 11-pound reduction dropped his pressure enough for his doctor to take him off the anti-hypertensive medication that had been prescribed.

Art's greatest obstacle to sticking with our program has been his long workdays, which often extend for ten hours or more. That doesn't leave much time for exercise, so Art has relied on low-fat eating as the mainstay of his plan. His wife, Carol, and daughter, Melissa, were part of the TODAY show volunteer group, too, and they have all been conscientious about avoiding high-fat foods.

Art doesn't let those lengthy workdays sabotage his low-fat eating. "It's virtually impossible for me to take a lunch hour, so I have to eat at my desk," he said. "I pack a lunch, and Carol makes sure healthy choices are available, like low-fat yogurt, fruit, bagels, and carrot sticks. They really hit the target of the fat content the program recommends."

Even so, Art's in-office lunches certainly aren't leisurely, so he finds it a challenge to concentrate on eating slowly and avoid the distractions of ringing phones and other inevitable interruptions. "I try to compensate by limiting the amount of food I take to work for lunch," he said. "Even if I eat faster than I should, I don't have a huge quantity of food with me so I'm able to limit the intake. Though the situation isn't perfect, I try to make it work."

There's another benefit to Art and Carol's low-fat commitment: They have five children, and many of their (and Melissa's) low-fat habits have rubbed off on the other kids. "Our youngest child went from whole milk down to skim, and won't drink anything else," he said. "Another child switched to 2% milk, which is what she prefers. They're even reading labels and becoming aware of the fat content of many foods."

In the best circumstances, Art takes a walk every day, and sometimes twice a day. But when the work demands become pressing, he has sometimes gone weeks with only sporadic exercise. Still, on a recent Saturday, Art awakened at 6 a.m., and walked four miles. "When I started this program, regular exercise was new to me. But it made me feel better and sleep better, and I'm looking forward to getting back to it on a regular basis." In the meantime, he said, healthy food choices are keeping him headed in the right direction weight-wise.

Week 5

Assignment

1. Decrease fat in your diet so it accounts for less than 20 percent of your total calories for the day. To accomplish this, increase your intake of foods that have 10 percent or less of their calories from fat, and cut back significantly on foods with 30 percent or more of their calories from fat.

2. Cover at least three miles each day (walking or running at any pace, continuously or in smaller segments), or substitute any equivalent activity.

3. Walk up at least four flights of stairs.

4. Eat your meals using the pacing system, pausing 30 seconds between each bite.

5. Eat at least three meals a day.

6. Using the Self-Monitoring charts, score yourself at the end of each day for goals accomplished.

7. To determine how much fat you can cut out of your diet without feeling deprived, try to reduce your fat intake to the point where fat accounts for only 10 percent or less of your total calories for the day. On that day, you will need to cut back even further on foods that contain more than 20 percent of their calories in the form of fat, and put even more emphasis on choosing foods that are under 10 percent.

WEEK 6

Success Principle #6

ENGAGING IN REGULAR PHYSICAL ACTIVITY

If I had to pick the single lifestyle change that most improves your chances of long-term weight loss, I would recommend that you increase your physical activity. That recommendation may not come as a surprise, since many studies have shown that exercise is a critical factor in maintaining weight loss. More surprising to you may be the types of exercise I'd suggest. While all physical activities are helpful, I prefer walking to running, stair climbing to using a Stairmaster, and low-intensity aerobics to high-intensity aerobics. Why? The preferred activities are easier to do than the alternatives, can be done without equipment, and are very effective.

In fact, when it comes to losing weight, my choices are probably more effective than their high-intensity cousins. Even fidgeting (random, purposeless activity) can use up as many as 800 calories per day. Walking three miles burns just as many calories as running three miles; it just takes a little longer. I can walk forever without getting tired and without any pain; my limit with running is four miles. Stairs are everywhere, but Stairmasters are hard to find. Besides, although I can walk five flights of stairs ten times, I don't have time to make ten separate trips to the gym, and I get worn out trying to do 50 consecutive flights.

I consider physical activity so essential to your long-term success—not only for weight loss, but also for fitness—that I strongly encourage you to continue it during the Continuity Phase, built around walking and stair climbing if those are the activities you choose to do. The point of our walking assignments has been to show you—gradually and safely—that anyone can exercise. Exercise doesn't have to hurt to be good for you, and it's almost as easy as walking out your front door. (In bad weather, you don't even have to go outside; cover the distance by walking in circles in your house.) Our stair-climbing exercise has been designed to remind you that stairs are made to be climbed, not avoided. Most of us have become expert at avoiding stairs. Now, we hope you are seeking them out and climbing them anytime you need to get to a higher floor.

The wide latitude you have been given in our plan—for the activities you can do, the time you can take, and the unlimited number of segments into which you can divide your exercise assignment—leaves you with almost no excuse for skipping exercise. Only a medical excuse will do. By the way, just because you are exercising doesn't mean you shouldn't keep looking for other ways to increase your physical activity each day. Whether that activity is purposeful (for instance, walking to the market instead of driving) or not (for example, walking in circles while you talk on the phone), it all counts toward weight loss.

Leading an Active Life: Bonnie Gonsalves

Bonnie Gonsalves has dieted most of her adult life, and exercise was sometimes part of those efforts. She'd join a health club, work out two or three times a week, but would never really lose any weight.

Things changed when Bonnie became part of our TODAY show group. She began walking seven days a week, and that seems to have made the difference in her ability to lose weight over the long haul.

"I try to walk four and a half miles a day," says Bonnie, who won't even let bad weather keep her indoors. "When it's hot, I walk early in the morning or late in the evening. And when it's raining, I bring an umbrella. I feel deprived if I can't take my walk."

The results: Bonnie lost 22 pounds in the first three months of the program, and at last report, was down a total of 25 pounds. "I feel great, and I believe the daily exercise is the reason."

Recently, Bonnie has even added some weight training and situps to her exercise routine. And how's this for commitment: When she vacationed recently in Northern California with her children, she visited an exercise equipment store and asked if she could do some repetitions on their workout stations. "I told them I couldn't pack my weights on the trip," said Bonnie, "and they said, 'Sure, help yourself!'" She did mini-workouts there twice that week.

Bonnie believes that her dedication to exercise gives her more flexibility in what she eats. "I stick with the low-fat eating guidelines almost all the time," she said, "but I can go out for Mexican food once in a while, and it doesn't affect my weight, as long as I'm exercising."

The daily exercise routine has made Bonnie much more thoughtful about the food she buys, because she knows how long it takes to walk off the excess fat calories. So she reads labels, and has made the switch to items like nonfat mayonnaise and sour cream. Her family has cut out red meat from their diet, and they eat more fruit, vegetables, rice, and pasta. Her children eat fat-free hot dogs, and instead of hamburgers, they enjoy lean ground turkey.

The exercise may have helped her control her appetite, too. "Overall, I eat a lot less food than I used to, and I get full faster," said Bonnie.

Bonnie's daily walks and her weight training are not her only avenues of exercise. "If I'm headed anywhere that has stairs—like going to my doctor's third floor office—I always make a point of taking the stairs. I don't look for close parking spaces, either, but instead park at the edge of the lot. You can fit in a lot of extra exercise that way."

Some of Bonnie's friends have suggested that she switch from walking to running, but thus far, she has resisted. "I love walking," she said. "And it doesn't take any special skill. You just put one foot in front of the other—and go!"

Week 6

Assignment

1. Decrease fat in your diet so it accounts for less than 20 percent of your total calories for the day. To accomplish this, increase your intake of foods that have 10 percent or less of their calories from fat, and cut back significantly on foods with 30 percent or more of their calories from fat.

2. Cover at least three miles each day (walking or running at any pace, continuously or in smaller segments), or substitute any equivalent activity.

3. Walk up at least four flights of stairs.

4. Eat your meals using the pacing system, pausing 30 seconds between each bite.

5. Eat at least three meals a day.

6. Using the Self-Monitoring charts, score yourself at the end of each day for goals accomplished.

7. To promote this week's Success Principle, commit yourself to try at least one new activity this week. You can do it as a substitute for walking or in addition to your walking assignment, but make it something different. Among the choices you should consider: ballroom dancing, square dancing, swimming, hiking, and biking.

WEEK 7

Success Principle #7

DEALING WITH STRESS

Life in the modern world involves high levels of stress. But you don't have to let stress make you sick or push you to eat to excess. That's exactly the way many people respond to stress, though—as I know from personal experience. Stress had been triggering my eating urges for at least two decades. My reactive eating got started during my first year of medical school—a time of marathon study sessions accompanied by world-class eating binges. Don't ask me why, but food made me feel better. It wasn't long before stress and food became inextricably intertwined for me, with the result that my weight ballooned up from 160 pounds to nearly 200.

I've known for years about the connection between stress and my overeating, but I couldn't get control of the situation until 1977. That's when I first learned about the value of relaxation techniques and started using them myself. Using these techniques regularly, I was able to reduce the ill feelings that stress produced and, consequently, my urge to eat. The situation improved even more when I added exercise to my daily routine. Exercise dramatically limited the tension and anxiety that stress produced and significantly reduced the frequency of my stress-triggered eating urges.

Now, I use both relaxation techniques and physical exercise to control the ill effects of stress. But I still often find myself feeling a little stressed or anxious when I sit down to eat. To keep these feelings from influencing me to overeat, I take a few deep breaths before each meal to calm myself down. That simple relaxation technique seems to interrupt the link in my mind between stress and food, and is usually all it takes to stop my reactive eating. I also end up feeling better.

Remember, the pacing program that you are using to focus your attention on eating begins with a simple breathing technique. Continue to use this simple technique before every meal, including snacks, to calm your mind and body, and to break any connection between stress and your urge to eat. The pacing program also contains a simple hunger test—a few questions that help you decide, in seconds, whether you are about to eat in response to real hunger, or are instead eating as a reaction to stress or some other psychological or emotional trigger. If you really are hungry, go ahead and eat. If not, try to find a more appropriate response to the feelings you are experiencing. Even three or four minutes will suffice to get you through the relaxation technique, the hunger test, and a few paced bites—enough, at least, to get you started eating your meal at the right speed.

Separating Stress from Eating: Helen Robinson

When life got stressful, Helen Robinson used to turn to food for comfort. Helen holds down two jobs to help support her family. If she became upset at work in the past, she might respond with emotional eating—reaching for a handful of potato chips or peanuts to soothe her anxiety.

But Helen reacts to stress differently now, and that has helped her lose weight and keep it off. She lost 22 pounds in the first three months of our program, and at last report, her total weight loss was 30 pounds.

Months after becoming part of the TODAY show volunteer group, Helen recognized that she now deals with stress differently. "When I get upset these days, it's very rare that I reach for food," she said. "I go out and do something more productive instead. I may go shopping and buy myself a new shirt or something else I want—other than food."

Today, Helen doesn't even keep "junk food" within reach. "My shopping patterns are completely different now," she said. "I don't buy cakes, cookies, and chips like I used to. Now, I keep rice cakes in my desk drawer at work, whereas in the past, you might have found peanuts."

Learning to respond differently to stress at work has helped Helen improve her food choices everywhere else.

"It's downright hard, because I like fried food," she said. "A restaurant just opened nearby that makes great French fries, and for me, that place is an accident waiting to happen! Or sometimes, I can see Twinkies dancing by, and I can hear them singing, 'Come on down to the kitchen, Helen . . .' But I've learned to abstain from those kinds of food, and I don't even keep them in my house anymore. I don't buy them to tempt me."

Getting control over simple things—like the snacks she keeps in her desk and her cupboard at home—makes Helen feel more in control of everything, and has increased the confidence she has in herself. If anyone doubts her new sense of self-assurance, they need only look at the way she dresses. "Last summer, I wore shorts a lot," she said. "I'm not a svelte size 8 or anything, but I sure feel more comfortable wearing shorts. Maybe it doesn't have as much to do with the weight loss as with my new attitude. I feel so much better, mentally and physically."

And what are her long-range goals? "My original goal was to lose 100 pounds, and that's still where I'm headed. I'm going to do it, even if it takes three years. No doubt about it."

THE STRESS SOURCE QUESTIONNAIRE

Here is a way to evaluate the effect of the stress in your life. For each of the potential sources of stress on the questionnaire, you will need to do the following:

a. Estimate how many times a week this source actually creates stress for you, and enter that number in the *Frequency* column.

b. Estimate how severe the stress is for each source based on the following scale, and enter that number in the *Degree* column:

   1 = only a little

   2 = annoying, but easily controlled

   3 = moderately severe (causes mild upset or discomfort)

   4 = severe (causes anxiety, irritability, anger, depression)

   5 = very severe (actually produces physical symptoms)

c. Estimate the total impact this has on your life each week by multiplying the number in the *Frequency* column by the number in the *Degree* column. Enter your answer in the *Impact* column.

STRESS SOURCE QUESTIONNAIRE

Sources of Stress   *Frequency*   *Degree*   *Impact*

RELATIONSHIPS

Spouse

Children

Parents

Other relatives

Friends

Neighbors

WORK

Boss

Coworkers

Job satisfaction

Environment

Lack of recognition

PERSONAL

Health problems

Self-image

Goals

Sex

FINANCIAL

Income

Expenses

Investments

Week 7

Assignment

1. Decrease fat in your diet so it accounts for less than 20 percent of your total calories for the day. To accomplish this, increase your intake of foods that have 10 percent or less of their calories from fat, and cut back significantly on foods with 30 percent or more of their calories from fat.

2. Cover at least three miles each day (walking or running at any pace, continuously or in smaller segments), or substitute any equivalent activity.

3. Walk up at least four flights of stairs.

4. Eat your meals using the pacing system, pausing 30 seconds between each bite.

5. Eat at least three meals a day.

6. Using the Self-Monitoring charts, score yourself at the end of each day for goals accomplished.

7. To enhance your efforts with this week's Success Principle, take a moment now to review the Stress Source Questionnaire on the preceding pages. Your answers will help you identify areas of your life that continue to produce stress. After reviewing the questionnaire, take time to develop some plans for dealing with those stressful areas.

WEEK 8

Success Principle #8
MONITORING YOUR ACTIVITIES

Weighing yourself on a scale, while important, will not provide you with the information you need to determine what weight-loss activities are working for you and what is still a problem. As in the 28-day program, you can continue to monitor and chart not only your weight, but also the activities you are doing to manage your weight. When your weight is dropping at a satisfactory rate, these charts will help you determine which activities are responsible for your success. If your weight is not responding as it should, the charts will help you identify areas in which you are having problems.

I find that these charts help me most when I display them prominently. I keep mine on the door in my office, where they remind me constantly of the good things I am doing for myself. I am also greatly motivated by the fact that my coworkers can see them, too. I recommend that you take these charts out of the book and post them in a place where you will see them several times a day. (If you prefer not to share your charts with others, keep them in your dresser drawer or in your car.) If it will motivate you, as it does me, to know that others can also monitor your progress, post your charts on the refrigerator door, next to your medicine cabinet, or at your workstation.

Your goal each day is not just to fill in circles on the chart, but to reflect on what those entries tell you about your weight management efforts. Just marking the charts doesn't make them useful; instead, what helps is analyzing your accomplishments and identifying which activities are working well for you and which are not.

Obesity is a chronic, lifelong condition. If excess weight has been a lifelong problem for you, I believe you should seriously consider continuing monitoring and charting your weight-management activities for the rest of your life. If that sounds like too much work, think of how much work would be involved in regaining and losing the same weight, over and over again, because you weren't willing to treat your weight problem as a chronic condition.

Charting the Way to Success: Scarlett Bates

Scarlett Bates has lost about 20 pounds on our weight-control program, and has maintained that success for many months. Yet like everyone, she has occasional moments when she backslides, sometimes without even realizing it. That's when closely monitoring her eating behavior and exercise habits pays off.

Scarlett leads a busy life as a legal secretary, and although she diligently charted her eating and exercise habits early in this program, she sometimes overlooked the record-keeping in more recent months. The charting, particularly when the program began, helped pave the way for her success, she said. It forced her to pay attention to the fat in the foods she chose. "After a while, I knew how much fat was in the foods I generally eat. Unless I eat something not normally on my personal menu, I have a good sense of the fat content of what's on my plate."

But Scarlett's early success with our program may have made her a little overconfident. At one point, as she stopped charting, the numbers on her scale gradually started to climb. Initially, she wasn't sure how to react. Now, if her weight goes up, she immediately returns to charting, monitoring the fat in her diet, her eating speed, and her activity level.

"If I gain four or five pounds, I generally can't identify on my own those areas that may have caused the problem," said Scarlett. "So I go back to charting to figure out exactly how I'm doing, and areas where I need to improve."

Charting helped Scarlett recognize that her biggest problem with eating occurred at work. "There are times when things become so busy at work that I'm not even aware of what I'm eating," she said. "I buy something at the vending machine without even realizing what I'm doing until I look back on the day and ask myself, 'What did I eat?' and 'Why did I eat it?'"

In addition to helping identify problems, Scarlett's charts have also become a source of great satisfaction—especially the exercise portion of the chart. When she sees all those exercise circles filled in, she remains somewhat astonished at her progress—and prowess—in this area. "Now, not only do I run three miles a day, but I'm also doing weight training three to four times a week, and I just took the certification exam to become a personal trainer." Not bad for someone who had never really been active before.

Week 8

Assignment

1. Decrease fat in your diet so it accounts for less than 20 percent of your total calories for the day. To accomplish this, increase your intake of foods that have 10 percent or less of their calories from fat, and cut back significantly on foods with 30 percent or more of their calories from fat.

2. Cover at least three miles each day (walking or running at any pace, continuously or in smaller segments), or substitute any equivalent activity.

3. Walk up at least four flights of stairs.

4. Eat your meals using the pacing system, pausing 30 seconds between each bite.

5. Eat at least three meals a day.

6. Using the Self-Monitoring charts, score yourself at the end of each day for goals accomplished.

7. To review the benefits of self-monitoring, take time this week to compare the charts you completed during the first two weeks of the program with the two most recent weeks' charts. Then answer these questions:

    a. During which period did you come closest to meeting your goals?

    b. Which is your strongest area now (cutting fat, physical activity, changing behavior)?

    c. Which is your weakest area now (cutting fat, physical activity, changing behavior)?

    d. What can you do to capitalize more on your strengths and minimize your weaknesses?

WEEK 9

Success Principle #9

BELIEVING IN AND CARING ABOUT YOURSELF

Too often, people who are obese have had their self-esteem undermined by their weight problem. They have stopped believing in and caring about themselves, largely because they have been unable to get their weight regulator under control.

As you read in Day 14 (page 182), your attitudes about yourself can significantly affect your ability to lose weight and keep it off. If you've been disappointed and felt guilty as you failed on one diet after another in recent years, it has probably taken a toll on your belief in yourself, and your sense that you are a worthwhile person.

I hope that in the first 28 days of this program, you have begun to care more about yourself, and started to separate your weight from your self-worth. Whether you are overweight or underweight, it should not affect your feelings about your own value as a human being. As this Continuity Phase evolves, allow your actions and thoughts to demonstrate an increasingly strong belief in yourself.

Making Yourself a Top Priority: Suzanne Kraft

Suzanne Kraft is a perfect example of how weight should be lost: slowly, steadily, and confidently. When we last spoke to her, nine months after she started the plan, she had lost a total of 44 pounds.

"I feel I have the tools now," Suzanne said with an air of confidence. She has a strong sense of self, and an ability—finally—to make her own well-being a top priority. As the mother of three and the grandmother of six, she spent most of her adult life caring for others, and food came to represent love in those family relationships. At the same time, however, food was Suzanne's poison, causing gains in weight that she could not successfully control.

"It's hard to learn to treat yourself with importance," said Suzanne. "Mothers, particularly, consider themselves the last ones who get attention." But she finally came to care enough about herself to tell her family, "I love you, and want to spend time with you over food, but it will have to be low-fat food." Fortunately, her family reacted with warmth and support.

Suzanne has also learned to be assertive about her nutritional needs outside the family setting—quite an achievement for someone who used to refrain from asking a waiter to divide a portion, concerned that it would cause him too much work. Now, when Suzanne dines out, she explains how she wants her seafood cooked, asks that the French fries be left in the kitchen, and insists that the salad dressing be placed on the side. When she accompanies her grandchildren to a fast-food restaurant, she orders a plain hamburger, and dresses it with tomatoes, lettuce, onions and pickles from the salad bar.

Suzanne starts every day now by taking care of herself. She is outdoors exercising by 6:00 a.m., sometimes earlier. She walks a mile to the grade school, and climbs and descends the stairs near the school a dozen times. Then she heads for the high school stadium, and walks 12 revolutions of the quarter-mile track. Finally, she heads for home, which adds another mile to her workout—for a total of five miles. All this at about the time the rest of the city is just beginning to stir.

But Suzanne is the first to tell you that her weight-loss efforts aren't easy. For so many years, she had a love affair with food, and that's a relationship that's hard to break. "For me, it's a constant battle, and I always have to be vigilant," she said.

Suzanne appreciates all that she's achieved thus far—not just losing weight, but caring more about herself, and comfortably putting her own health needs up there with everyone else's. "I've made wonderful progress on this program," she said, "and I continue to recommend it to others."

Week 9

Assignment

1. Decrease fat in your diet so it accounts for less than 20 percent of your total calories for the day. To accomplish this, increase your intake of foods that have 10 percent or less of their calories from fat, and cut back significantly on foods with 30 percent or more of their calories from fat.

2. Cover at least three miles each day (walking or running at any pace, continuously or in smaller segments), or substitute any equivalent activity.

3. Walk up at least four flights of stairs.

4. Eat your meals using the pacing system, pausing 30 seconds between each bite.

5. Eat at least three meals a day.

6. Using the Self-Monitoring charts, score yourself at the end of each day for goals accomplished.

7. To put this week's Success Principle into practice, do something nice for yourself this week. Reward yourself for your persistence and success. The reward doesn't have to be expensive, but it should be meaningful to you: Buy yourself a book; take a friend to a movie; or schedule a weekend treat.

WEEK 10

Success Principle #10

CREATING YOUR SUPPORT NETWORK

Since the start of the 28-day program, I hope you have found a network of friends and family members who can offer you support during the weeks and months ahead. They can provide encouragement if you backslide a little, and pats on the back when you're doing well. They can help you troubleshoot when you're having problems, and celebrate as you reach your weight-loss goals. They can become your walking partners, and help you prepare low-fat meals in your kitchen (or theirs).

If you haven't yet established a support network for yourself, refer back to Day 10 (page 165) for suggestions on how to get started. During times when your self-motivation wanes a little, a support system can help you stay on track.

A Family Support System: Susan Lydon

When Susan Lydon sought a support system for her current weight-loss efforts, she looked no further than her own family. Susan's father, Ed, had actually talked her into joining the TODAY show group, and they've turned to each other for encouragement and support ever since.

"We try to eat lunch together once a week, and we talk on the phone often about how we're doing," said Susan. That support has helped her lose weight steadily. She dropped about a pound a week in the first three months—a total decline of 12 pounds—and increased that loss to a total of 15 pounds after six months. At the nine-month point, she was down 23 pounds.

"My father has not only been supportive, but he's very inspirational, too," said Susan. "He's dealt with a weight problem most of his life, and this is the first time that he's really embraced exercise as a component of an overall weight-loss program. It's had a dramatic and positive impact on his overall health."

Susan has found this program different than others she has tried. "It's really a way of life," she said. "With other programs, you go in and they tell you what to eat, and you weigh in once a week. But this time, I've learned to make my own healthy choices involving food and exercise for the rest of my life. It's not only been easier to adopt, but more important, easier to maintain."

Four to five times a week, Susan runs or walks briskly for three to four miles, either outdoors or on a treadmill. As she tells her father during their informal "support group" lunches, regular exercise is the most important element of her program. "Yes, I eat slower and eat less, and make good food choices," she said. "But I think exercise is what has kept the weight loss going, and has changed my body shape."

Many of Susan's friends have been supportive, too, commenting frequently on the positive changes in her physical appearance. "I have a completely different figure," she said. "My body shape has changed so much in terms of the size of clothes I wear and the way they look on me. I really attribute this to exercise."

When the temperature rose during the summer, Susan admits it was sometimes hard to muster the energy to exercise. At one point, she didn't work out for two weeks, and could feel the difference in a lot of ways. When her physical activity stopped, she also made some unhealthy food choices—but shortly after a conversation with her dad, she decided to get back on track. Once she began exercising again, the rest of the program fell back into place.

When Susan and her father signed on for this weight-loss effort, she recalled, their interests were quite different. She was most interested in achieving cosmetic benefits from her weight loss ("I wanted to look better"), while her dad was much more focused on improving his health. But since she's seen her father's health improve, she's been motivated to enhance her own physical well-being, too.

"I feel better physically, and I have more energy," said Susan. And that reinforcement is helping her stick with it—and continue to lose weight.

Week 10

Assignment

1. Decrease fat in your diet so it accounts for less than 20 percent of your total calories for the day. To accomplish this, increase your intake of foods that have 10 percent or less of their calories from fat, and cut back significantly on foods with 30 percent or more of their calories from fat.

2. Cover at least three miles each day (walking or running at any pace, continuously or in smaller segments), substituting any equivalent activity.

3. Walk up at least four flights of stairs.

4. Eat your meals using the pacing system, pausing 30 seconds between each bite.

5. Eat at least three meals a day.

6. Using the Self-Monitoring charts, score yourself at the end of each day for goals accomplished.

7. Put this week's Success Principle into practice by letting me join your support group. I really want to know how you are doing with this program, and I'd like you to feel that I am part of your support system. All you have to do is write to me. Let me know how you're doing, and send me your comments and suggestions for future editions of this book. You can write to me at the following address:

> Art Ulene, M.D.
> P.O. Box 7775
> Burbank, CA 91510-7775

The Next Step

At the pace of losing about one pound a week, the Continuity Phase of this program should have helped you move closer to your weight-loss goal in the past ten weeks. If you still have more pounds to lose, stick with the Continuity Phase in the weeks ahead, following the assignments in Week 10 indefinitely and enjoying your continuing loss of weight. By making wise choices in what you put on your plate, by eating at a slow pace, and by making exercise part of your daily schedule, your weight will keep decreasing until you're right where you want to be.

Once you finally reach your weight-loss objective, whether that's in a week or a year, then it's time to congratulate yourself on your achievement—and move on to the Maintenance Phase of the program. We haven't forgotten about one of the most important phases of any weight-loss plan—how to keep those lost pounds off for good. So when the time arrives to move from weight loss to weight maintenance, turn the page and find out how to enjoy permanent success.

12

THE MAINTENANCE PHASE

You have now reached your goal weight and are ready to begin the Maintenance Phase of the program. You should start by congratulating yourself. After many weeks (perhaps months) on this program, you finally weigh what you want to, and you should be proud of your accomplishment.

If you had been following a typical diet plan to lose the weight, it would now be time to quit the diet—which means, of course, that you'd start gaining the weight back. But this program is different from the diet plans you've tried in the past. Those diets treat obesity as if it were a short-term problem that can be cured simply by losing pounds. As you have already learned, however, the tendency to gain weight is a lifelong problem, and the only way to keep the weight off is with lifestyle changes that can be maintained for life.

Beginning in the first 28 days of this program, you learned what changes were necessary to lose weight, and you saw how those changes could become a natural—and permanent—part of your behavior and lifestyle. As you begin the Maintenance Phase you will continue these changes, but with some minor adjustments.

Adjustments to Make During the Maintenance Phase

Here are the adjustments you need to make during the Maintenance Phase, so that your new behaviors will work even more effectively over the long term.

Change the way you think about yourself. For years, you've probably pictured yourself as an overweight person. If, like many other people, you repeatedly lost weight and gained it back, you may also have seen yourself as out of control, irresponsible or inadequate (or, as many have said to me, all of the above).

But you've proven now that you can make healthy choices about food and exercise, and you've proven your ability to manage your weight. So it's time to recognize the progress you've made; it's time to change that overly critical image of yourself. Now that you've reached your target weight, one of the most important changes you can make is in the way you think about yourself. More than ever, you now have a reason to believe in yourself. So, do it!

Change the way others see you. Since the start of this program, you've been requesting support from family and friends in your weight-loss efforts. Now, as you enter the Maintenance Phase, their support is still important. But it's also crucial that these people begin to see you as a healthy person who is trying to stay that way, not as an overweight person attempting to shed pounds.

If family and friends keep referring back to their old overweight image of you, gently correct these old impressions. Keep in mind that you'll need their support for the rest of your life to maintain the progress you've made. But don't be afraid to ask them to acknowledge that progress, too. Their change in attitude will help you to maintain a healthier and more current picture of yourself.

Weigh yourself daily. For years, the scale has probably been your enemy. However, in the Maintenance Phase, the scale becomes one of your strongest allies, because it can warn you early if you

FINDING SUPPORT IN YOUR LIFE

Even though you no longer need to lose weight, it's still nice to have continuing support for the Maintenance Phase. Many of our TODAY show participants—some of whom have already reached their weight-loss goals—still meet informally, recognizing the value of sharing and discussing how they're doing. "We have so much fun when we get together," Helen Robinson says. "Everyone brings a low-fat dish, and we talk about how we've been doing. We laugh a lot, support each other, and the sharing helps keep us going."

start drifting off your plan. From now on, you should start weighing yourself every day (though not more than once a day). Daily weighing is not done to add more emphasis to your weight, but to help you catch problems before you stray too far off course.

There is no need to panic if your weight varies by a pound or two on any given day. After all, something as simple as a high-sodium meal or an approaching menstrual period can make a person gain that much weight just through water retention. Your weight will even vary from one time of the day to another (it's almost always higher at night, after dinner, than early in the morning, before breakfast). These minor weight shifts due to water retention are temporary, and will correct themselves.

If your weight rises three or more pounds, however, you need to ask: "Why have I gained this weight, and what adjustments do I need to make in my choice of foods, my activity level, or my eating behaviors?" The faster you make these adjustments, the less likely you are to become discouraged and drift even farther from your goal weight. If you've gained five or six pounds, then it's time to restart the detailed daily monitoring of fat intake, exercise, and eating speed that enabled you to lose the weight earlier. The daily charting will help you identify problems more quickly. Also, as you have probably already discovered, the charting makes you stick more closely to your plan.

Switch from a "low-fat" to a "high-health" diet. When this weight-loss plan began, I asked you to switch to a low-fat diet. As you start the Maintenance Phase, it's time to switch again—this time, to a "high-health" diet of foods that are brimming with complex carbohydrates, fiber, vitamins, and minerals.

Is this really a change in the way you are already eating? No. These nutrient-rich foods are almost always naturally low in fat. But what I'm suggesting is a change in your attitude and approach, from the negative (*avoid fats*) to the positive (*seek out delicious foods that are really good for you*). I believe that this small shift in focus makes it easier and more fun to maintain your new lifestyle (and your new weight) on a lifelong basis.

FINDING A HEALTHIER LIFESTYLE

Bonnie Gonsalves, one of our TODAY show volunteers, says, "Once I made the switch to healthier, lower-fat foods, it became a habit. In fact, it has actually become easy. My entire family has become very aware of which foods are healthier than others. We've decided to make many of these dietary changes together."

Pay even closer attention to the sensory qualities of the food you eat. You've already learned how important it is to stay attentive to what and how you're eating when you are losing weight—especially your eating speed. Most people say this is the most difficult part of our program to learn. Unfortunately, it is also one of the easiest parts to forget. Whenever you lower your guard, your lifetime habits tend to creep back in. Eating speed is no exception.

So, how do you maintain your slower eating pace without timing every bite? By taking time to enjoy the flavor of your food; by taking time to enjoy the aroma of your food; by taking time to enjoy the consistency of your food. The more you concentrate on these sensory pleasures, the less you'll have to think about your eating speed. That will take care of itself.

Some Things Should Stay the Same

Some of the things you did to lose weight should not be changed now that you've moved into the Maintenance Phase of the program. These activities will remain effective for a lifetime.

Make physical activity a daily part of your life. Exercise is often the first component of the program to be dropped when people reach their goal weight and begin the Maintenance Phase. For reasons that are difficult to explain (I blame it on the weight regulator), some individuals who worked so hard to get their weight down suddenly decide they can keep it down without any effort. This kind of thinking ignores the fact that a malfunctioning weight regulator stays stuck on its high set point for life.

To maintain your new weight, it is essential that you continue to lead a physically active lifestyle, not only exercising on a daily basis, but taking advantage of every opportunity to increase your "ordinary" activity (like climbing stairs or walking to the market). Even small incremental increases in physical activity can have big payoffs in helping you maintain your weight loss over the long term. It's tempting to believe you can get away without exercise during the Maintenance Phase, and there will be many reasons—such as a shortage of time—that will make you think about skipping some exercise sessions. Don't make that mistake. Once exercise goes, the rest of your program will quickly go, too. When that happens, it will not be long before your weight begins to climb.

Don't use food to manage stress. Even though you've reached your ideal weight, there will still be occasions when you feel like

FINDING JOY IN EATING

One of the men who uses our program in Berryville, Virginia, says that paying close attention to how he eats and the qualities of the food he's eating has changed his life. "I've gone from eating two and a half plates of food at every dinner down to one," he said. "But the real benefit is in the pleasure of eating. I never knew food could taste this good."

FINDING TIME FOR EXERCISE

If Helen Robinson were looking for an excuse to avoid physical activity, she wouldn't have to look far. She works two jobs and is raising a family, so she has difficulty just finding daytime hours when she can walk. But that hasn't stopped Helen from exercising.

Helen understands that exercise is critical to her success with this program. When she isn't able to get in her early morning walks, she jumps on an exercise bicycle at home in the evening. "I started out doing a half-mile on the exercise bike, and it was hard," she said. "But now, I've worked up to three miles a day, and I feel great." Helen looks great, too. After nine months on our program, she has lost 30 pounds and is steadily progressing toward her final goal weight.

reaching for food to comfort yourself or to relieve feelings of stress. With the passage of time, these feelings will probably strike you less frequently and with less strength. Nevertheless, you can expect them to keep popping up the rest of your life, so you must always be prepared to deal with them.

Two parts of your new eating "ritual" will help you overcome these urges: The brief relaxation technique and the hunger test. It is important that you continue to use the relaxation technique every time you eat, calming your mind and body before taking the first bite. And you should continue to use the hunger test before every bite, asking yourself each time: *"Am I really hungry, or is it something else I am feeling?"* (To refresh your memory on how to use these techniques, see page 113.) These two techniques will let you continue eating anytime you are hungry, but they will help you avoid those unsatisfying and guilt-provoking episodes of reactive or emotional eating. They will also help you maintain your goal weight.

A Closing Message

In the months and years ahead, your malfunctioning weight regulator will continue its efforts to push your weight back to its former level. Your new lifestyle can be a powerful force in resisting

FINDING OTHER STRESS RELIEVERS

Scarlett Bates tends to be an emotional eater. "But now when I feel like reaching for food in response to stress, I write in my journal instead," she says. "I make journal entries once a week, sometimes more often. It helps me put things in perspective, and keeps me from using food to combat stress."

those efforts. The key to long-term success? Never become complacent! If you begin to ignore any component of this program, your new state of well-being could be endangered.

Although this book and its day-by-day assignments are about to end, *your* plan for good health is just beginning. The general strategies I've described throughout the book can continue to help you for the rest of your life. But your long-term success depends on your making them *your* strategies and on developing *your own* action plans from now on.

I urge you now to take over the ownership of this program—to make a lifetime commitment to the pursuit of good health. If you do, you should never have to worry about excess weight again.

My best wishes to you for good health always.

Art Ulene, M.D.

RESOURCES

Dr. Art Ulene's Low-Fat Cookbook offers more information on low-fat cooking and recipes. You can order the cookbook by calling 1-800-428-4488.

Exercise à la Carte by Dr. George L. Dixon is available by calling 1-800-624-4952.

Secrets of Fat-Free Baking by Sandra Woodruff, RD, published by Avery Publishing Group, Inc. is available in bookstores everywhere, or can be ordered directly from the publisher by calling 1-800-548-5757.

INDEX

Accu-Measure, and body fat, 216

Activity program. *See* Exercise

Aerobic exercise, 47, 92–97, 143

Aerobics classes, 96

Affirmations, in pacing program, 112, 120–23

Age, and weight loss, 28

Alcohol, 200, 205–206

Appetite
 and dietary fat, 40
 and exercise, 38, 46

Appetizers, 169

Arthritis, and weight loss, 29

Averaging fat intake, 85–89, 285

Baking, 185–88

Bathroom scales, 182–83, 311–12

Beef, fat content, 130, 131

Behavior modification techniques, 52–56, 196–97. *See also* Pacing program

Behavioral changes in eating, 52–56, 107–23, 196–97

Bioelectrical impedance analysis, and body fat, 217

Biological factors, and obesity, 18–23

Body fat, 214–17
 and weight loss, 35–38
 weight of, 37–38

Body size, and metabolism, 21

Brain chemicals, 20

Breakfast, 170, 226

Butter, fat content, 135–36

Calories
 banking, 222–23
 burned during exercise, 95
 calculating percentage from fat, 128–29
 counting, 39–41, 285
 density, 42–43, 138
 from fat, 39–40, 128–29, 285–86
 in serving size, 128

Cancer, 41, 78

Carbohydrates, 42, 202–203

Case studies
 using progress charts, 258–66
 using self-monitoring charts, 63–73

Celebrations, and eating, 199–200

Cereals, 126

Changes, small, 147–48, 180, 229, 231–32, 273

importance of, 26–27

See also Substitutes

Charts

importance of, 299–301

progress type, 247–66

self-monitoring type, 59–73

Cheese, fat content, 133–34, 135

Chicken, fat content, 130, 131, 132–33

Chinese food, 171

Chips, 210–11

Cholesterol, and fat in diet, 41, 78

"Cholesterol-free" on food labels, 127

Cigarette smoke, 21

Clothing, for exercise, 192, 193

Cognitive change, and behavior modification, 55

Complex carbohydrates, 202–203

Conditioning Phase, 81, 83–240

steps, 83–84

Continuity Phase, 81, 234, 241–309

success principles, 268–309

Cookies, 211

nonfat, 126

Cooking, 232

Cooking methods, 158–59. *See also* Food preparation

Cookware, 158, 232

Cross-country ski stimulators, 96–97

Cycling, 96

Dairy products, fat content, 133–36

Dairy substitutes, 186, 187

Dancing, 162

Dark/light meat, 132–33

Desserts

fat content, 137

in restaurants, 172–73

DEXA, and body fat, 217

Diabetes, as disease, 11, 15–16

Dietary fat *See* Fat in diet

Diets and dieting,

failure of, and weight loss, 29–30

traditional, 12–13, 25–26, 78

Dining out, 169–73, 225–26

Distances, estimating, 140–42

Dixon, George, 161

Drugs, and weight loss, 11, 16–17

Eating

behaviors, 276–78

modifying behavior, 196–97, 52–56, 107–23, 196–97

as sensory pleasure, 313

speed, 107–23, 212, 276–78, 313

Eggs, 170

Emotional issues, and eating, 150–56

Endorphins, 20, 78

Environmental issues, and obesity, 23–24

Ethnic foods, 171

Exercise, 22, 45–51, 140–45, 289–91, 293

aerobic, 47, 92–97, 143

alternatives, 161–63

commitment, 48–49

and Conditioning Phase, 91–105
equivalents, 142–45
excuses for skipping, 190–94
finding time for, 178–80
and Maintenance Phase, 314, 315
and medical checkup, 50
and metabolism, 46
and strength training, 47–48, 97–104
See also Fitness
Exercise bicycles, 96–97
Exercise videotapes, 97

Family support, and weight loss, 30, 165–67, 306–307, 311, 312
Fast-food meals, 225–26
Fat
added to food, 231–32
calculating percentage in diet, 128–29
cells, 20
"counter" books, 285–86
in diet, 39–44, 85–89, 128–29, 284–87
storage, 20–21
Fat-free foods, 134
and food labels, 127, 231
Fiber, 203
Fidgeting, 22, 289
Fish, fat content, 130, 131, 132
Fitness, 77–82, 237–38
vs. weight loss, 244–45
See also Exercise
Food
alternatives. *See* Substitutes
diaries, 58

extenders, 175
labels, 125–29, 231
preparation, 158–59, 185–88, 232
See also specific foods
Frank, Arthur, 10–11, 14
French food, 171
Fried foods, 158
Fruit substitutes, for fat, 186–87

Gender, and weight loss, 28–29
Genetic factors, and weight problems, 18, 19
Goals
realistic, 238, 239, 243–44
weekly, 246–47
Ground meats, fat content, 131, 133
Guilt, 237

Health, and lifestyle changes, 78–79
Health benefits, of low-fat diet, 41
Heart disease, and fat in diet, 78
Heart rate, maximum, 92, 144–45, 238
Heredity, and obesity, 18, 19
High blood pressure
as disease, 11, 16
and weight loss, 78–79
High-fat foods, 129–37
alternatives, 42–43
See also Substitutes
High-fat ingredients, for baking, 187
Hormones, 22–23
Hunger monitoring, 155–56
Hunger pangs, 110

Hunger test, in pacing program, 110, 113

Hypertension, as disease, 11, 16

Ice cream, fat content, 137

Illness, and weight loss, 29

Insulin, 15–16

Italian food, 171

Japanese food, 171

Jogging, 94

Labels, food. *See* Food, labels

Lapses in program, 280–82

"Law of averages," and fat intake, 85–89, 285

"Lean" on food labels, 127

Leptin, and obesity, 19

Life expectancy, and fitness level, 78

Lifestyle changes, benefits, 78–79

"Light" ("lite") on food labels, 127, 231

Light/dark meat, 132–33

Lipoprotein lipase, 20–21

Liquid sweeteners, 186, 188

Liquor, 200, 205–206

Low-fat diets, 41, 284–87

"Low-fat" on food labels, 127

Low-fat foods, 134–35, 229–31, 233

Maintenance Phase, 82, 234, 310–16

Margarine, fat content, 135–36

Maximum heart rate, 92, 144–45, 238

Meals, skipping, 111

Meat, fat content, 130, 131

Medical checkup, before exercising, 50

Men, and weight loss, 28–29

Metabolism, 21

change in, 293

and exercise, 46

and skipping meals, 111

Mexican food, 171

Milk, fat content, 133, 135

Monitoring. *See* Self-monitoring program

Motivation, and weight loss, 28

Muscle tissue, 35–38

loss of, 35–37

tone, 37, 38, 143

weight of, 37–38

Nonstick spray, 232

Nutritional labels. *See* Food, labels

Obesity

and degree of weight loss, 29

as disease, 10, 16–17

duration of, and weight loss, 29

and exercise, 49–50

gene, 19

Oils, fat content, 136

Osteoporosis, 214

and exercise, 78

Pacing program, 108–23, 276–78, 294

affirmations, 112, 120–23

hunger test, 110, 113

pacing system, 110-11, 113–19

relaxation exercise, 109–10, 113

script, 113–23

Pacing system, in pacing program, 110–11, 113–19

Parties, and eating, 199–200

Patience, importance of, 272–74

Pedometers, 142

"Percent Daily Value" on food labels, 129

Percentage of calories from fat, 85–89, 128–29, 285

Physical activity. *See* Exercise

Pickles, 138

Plan, importance of, 268–70

Plateaus, in weight loss, 208

Portion size. *See* Serving size

Potatoes, 225–26

Poultry, fat content, 130, 131, 132–33

Pretzels, 126, 138

Progress charts, 247–57
    case studies, 258–66

Psychological issues
    and eating, 150–56
    and obesity, 23

Psychotherapy, 154

Pulse rate, 92, 144–45, 238
    measuring, 144–45

Reactive eating, 150–56
    questionnaire, 153

Reinforcement, and behavior modification, 55

Relaxation exercise, in pacing program, 109–10, 113

Relaxation techniques, 293

Responsibility, personal, 245–46

Restaurant meals, 169–73, 225–26

Resting metabolic rate (RMR). *See* Metabolism

Rowing machines, 96–97

Running, 94

Sabotage efforts, of family and friends, 166–67

Salad bars, 225

Salad dressings, 170
    fat content, 136

Sandwiches, 170, 212

Script, for pacing program, 113–23

Seafood, fat content, 130, 131, 132

Self-assessment questionnaire, 235–39

Self-image, 311

Self-monitoring program, 57–74
    and behavior modification, 54–55
    case studies, 63–73
    charts, 59–62
    problems, common, 63–73

Self-worth, 182–83, 303–304

Sensory pleasures, of eating, 313

Serotonin inhibitors, 154

Serving size, 125–28, 130, 138, 228–29
    in restaurants, 172

Set point, 10, 16, 17–18

Setbacks in program, 280–82

Sex. *See* Gender

Skin-fold measurement, and body fat, 216

Skipping meals, 111

Smoking, 21

Snacks and snacking, 210–12
    fat content, 137, 138

Soups, 170, 212

Stair climbing, 105, 162, 289–90

Stair climbing machines, 96–97

Stationary exercise machines, 96–97

Stimulus control, and behavior modification, 53–54

Strength training, 47–48, 97–104

Stress, 293–95
  and Maintenance Phase, 314–15, 316

Stress source questionnaire, 296–97

Stride length, 141–42

Substitutes, 26, 175–76, 185–88
  in restaurants, 169, 170
  snacks, 210–12
  tables, 176, 187, 231, 232, 273
  when baking, 185–88

Success principles, of Continuity Phase, 268–309

Support groups and systems, 30, 165–67, 306–307, 311, 312

Swimming, 94, 96

Thermogenesis, 21–22

Three-ounces-a-day plan, 147–48

Thyroid, 22–23

TODAY show, 2–4

"Total Fat" on food labels, 129

Treadmills, 96–97

Turkey, fat content, 130, 131, 132–33

Ulene, Art, as support system address, 308

Underwater weighing, and body fat, 215–16

Vegetables, fat content, 138

Vegetarian diets, 42

Walking, 93–94, 144, 161, 162, 289–90
  and estimating distances, 140–42

Water aerobics, 94, 96

Water exercises, 94, 96

Water retention, 312

Water walking, 94

Weekly goals, and Continuity Phase, 246–47

Weighing self, 182–83, 311–12
  underwater, 215–16

Weight loss
  and fitness, 77–79
  gradual, 272–74
  rate, 219–20, 239, 241–42
  setbacks, 280–82

Weight regulator, 11, 15–24, 219–20, 242
  definition, 17
  and emotional and psychological issues, 151
  and exercise, 193
  overriding, 25–31, 41

Weight training. *See* Strength training

Weight-lifting equipment, 98

Well-being, sense of, 38

Willpower, 151, 155

Wine, 205

Women, and weight loss, 28–29

Woodruff, Sandra, 185

Yogurt, fat content, 134–35, 137, 211

Dear Reader:

Since we published our first weight-loss book, we've received thousands of inquiries from people who wanted a longer program to follow until they reach their goal weight. This new and greatly expanded book was designed to help meet their needs. However, many people—particularly those who have large amounts of weight to lose—want even more structure than a book can offer. In response to their requests, we have developed a program that delivers new materials on a monthly basis to subscribers' homes. Each shipment will include several of the following items:

- Weekly plans with detailed daily assignments
- Weekly charts for continued self-monitoring
- Computer-generated weight-loss projections that are customized for your starting weight, goal weight, age, gender, and activity level
- Monthly feedback forms for reporting your progress to me
- Telephone cards that give you access to daily updates, motivational messages, and "live" support sessions
- Low-fat recipes and cookbooks
- Exercise videos
- Audio and video motivational tapes

If you need extra help to achieve your weight goal, complete and **return the subscription form on the next page** or call **1-800-948-5677** to sign up today.

I look forward to hearing from you.

Art Ulene, M.D.

SUBSCRIPTION FORM

Name: _____

Address: _____

City: _____ State: _____ Zip: _____

Phone: (   )   (   )
               (day)   *(evening)*

YES, sign me up for Dr. Ulene's continuing program to help me reach my weight goal. I understand that the program includes monthly communication from the doctor.

Here is my first monthly payment of $29.95 (plus $4.95 shipping and handling—for a total of $34.90). I understand that I may cancel my subscription at any time. Mail this form with payment to HealthPOINTS, P.O. Box 407, Bridgewater, VA 22812.

Method of payment:
Check or money order, payable to HealthPOINTS

VISA❑ Mastercard❑ American Express❑   Exp. date: _____

Card No: _____ Date: _____

Signature:_____

Please allow 4-6 weeks for shipping. If for any reason you are not completely satisfied, you may return your shipment for a full refund—no questions asked.

LOSE WEIGHT AND FEEL GREAT!

Safe, effective weight-loss programs that take the weight off!

Get with the program and ditch those diet plans! This special program shows you how to lose weight naturally and safely! Discover how changing your eating pace, cutting out fat, and increasing activity can help you lose weight.

LOSE WEIGHT WITH DR. ART ULENE

Lose Weight with Dr. Art Ulene provides an excellent 28-day weight-loss program. Discover how participants across America followed the program and lost weight! Learn how to change your eating patterns, increase activity levels and have fun while losing weight!
VHS Video
Item No. V048 $19.95

STOP DIET DEPRESSION!

Learn how to control your eating habits and start feeling good about yourself!

LOSE WEIGHT NATURALLY

Eliminate the stress that comes from losing weight! Do it the relaxing, sensible way! Use this innovative "pacing" technique to help you control how much and how fast you eat. You'll also get a variety of positive affirmations to help you gain control and feel good about yourself! Plus, a 40-page booklet filled with tips and techniques for success!
Audio cassette & booklet.
Item No. A002 $14.95

EAT LESS FAT, NOT LESS FOOD!

Get the skinny on healthy, low-fat eating! End starvation diets forever! Give up starving yourself or skipping meals because you're afraid of weight gain. Just cut out the fat and presto! you'll watch the weight melt away. Discover how to prepare healthy, low-fat meals and snacks that taste great! You'll get all kinds of tips on how to eliminate the fat from your favorite foods and still have great tasting meals!
VHS video.
Item No. V021 $19.95

SLOW DOWN, SLIM DOWN

Slow down the pace and speed up your weight loss! Control the amount you eat by recognizing how fast you eat it! You'll savor the relaxation exercises and the pacing system that help you lose weight and increase the pleasure you get from eating. Plus, positive affirmations to help you develop the "I can do it" attitude!
VHS video.
Item No. V023 $14.95

GET FIT & STAY FIT!

Programs designed to work out the problems and work in a new you!

Get the most mileage out of your fitness program. The following programs are designed for people of all fitness levels. Stretch it out, tone it up, and work it out! You'll feel great!

TAMILEE WEBB'S BALANCED FITNESS WORKOUT

Stretch it, flex it, and tone it up! A flexible workout program designed to shape you up the safe, effective way. Part one warms you up, stretches you out, and cools you down. Part two gets the heart rate up with some fun aerobics designed to build flexibility and strength. It's simple and fun!
VHS video.
Item No. V006 $19.95

TAMILEE WEBB'S BODYBAND WORKOUT

Get on the band wagon and build that resistance! This fun workout uses bodybands to tone, stretch, and increase flexibility. Great for men and women! Bodybands are lightweight and easy to use—you can even take them with you when you travel! You'll look good and feel great!
Bonus! With the purchase of each *Bodyband Workout* video you get three bodybands and an informative booklet complete with do's and don'ts!
VHS video.
Item No. V005 $19.95

SPECIAL OFFER

Save $10! Purchase both tapes for a complete fitness program for only $29.90.
Balanced Fitness & Bodyband Package
Item No. K003 $29.90

DR. ART ULENE'S FITNESS WALKING PROGRAM

Get with the program and walk your way to healthier living! It's your walking papers and audio cassette in one neat package! This is absolutely one of the safest, most enjoyable fitness programs you can get your hands on! Benefit from a walking program that includes stretching, warming-up, a heart-healthy aerobic "walk-out" and cool-down. The audio tapes set the pace with music that gets you into step. Plus, an 80-page booklet gives you tips and techniques for maximum benefits and a handy log to chart your progress. Don't walk away from this one! Audio cassette & booklet.
Item No. A014 $14.95

FITNESS WALKING PROGRAM AND PEDOMETER

Track those miles with this handy pedometer ($25 retail value!) to go along with your audio and booklet! Save $5!
Audio & booklet with pedometer.
Item No. K004 $34.95

DR. ART ULENE'S NUTRIBASE NUTRITION FACTS DESK REFERENCE

Over 40,000 products and their nutrition values in one place! Find out exactly what you're eating! Get the first-hand facts on nutritional values of over 40,000 foods. Ever wonder what that fast food burger contains? Or that handful of trail mix? Find out with this "A to Z" reference book. Three comprehensive sections cover nutrients, vitamins, and minerals for some of America's best-loved foods! Use it to reference calories, fat content, and more! Book, softbound.
Item No. B006 $17.95

To order these books, audios, and videos call 800-697-9910 or write to HealthPOINTS, P.O. Box 407, Bridgewater, VA 22812. Include $4.95 for shipping and handling. California, Indiana, and Virginia residents, please add sales tax.

OTHER ULYSSES PRESS
HEALTH BOOKS

COUNT OUT CHOLESTEROL
Art Ulene, M.D. and Val Ulene, M.D.

Complete with counter and detailed dietary plan, this companion resource to the *Count Out Cholesterol Cookbook* shows how to design a cholesterol-lowering program that's right for you. $12.95

COUNT OUT CHOLESTEROL COOKBOOK
Art Ulene, M.D. and Val Ulene, M.D.

A companion guide to *Count Out Cholesterol*, this book shows you how to bring your cholesterol levels down with the help of 250 gourmet recipes. $14.95

THE VITAMIN STRATEGY
Art Ulene, M.D. and Val Ulene, M.D.

A game plan for good health, this book helps readers design a vitamin and mineral program tailored to their individual needs. $11.95

DISCOVERY PLAY
Art Ulene, M.D. and Steven Shelov, M.D.

This book guides parents through the first three years of their child's life, offering play activity with a special emphasis on nurturing self-esteem. $9.95

LAST WISHES: A HANDBOOK TO
GUIDE YOUR SURVIVORS
Lucinda Page Knox, M.S.W. and Michael D. Knox, Ph.D.

A simple do-it-yourself workbook, *Last Wishes* helps people put their affairs in order and eases the burden on their survivors. It allows them to plan their own funeral and leave final instructions for survivors. $12.95

IRRITABLE BOWEL SYNDROME: A NATURAL APPROACH
Rosemary Nicol

> This book offers a natural approach to a problem millions of sufferers have. The author clearly defines the symptoms and provides a dietary and stress-reduction program for relieving the effects of this disease. $9.95

KNOW YOUR BODY: THE ATLAS OF ANATOMY
Introduction by Trevor Weston, M.D.

> Designed to provide a comprehensive and concise guide to the structure of the human body, *Know Your Body* offers more than 250 color illustrations. An easy-to-follow road map of the human body. $11.95

PANIC ATTACKS: A NATURAL APPROACH
Shirley Trickett

> Addresses the problem of panic attacks using a holistic approach. With a simple program focusing on diet, breathing, and relaxation, the book helps you understand this phenomenon and teaches how to prevent future attacks. $8.95

BREAKING THE AGE BARRIER: STAYING YOUNG, HEALTHY AND VIBRANT
Helen Franks

> Drawing on the latest medical research, *Breaking the Age Barrier* explains how the proper lifestyle can stop the aging process and make you feel youthful and vital. $12.95

To order these or other Ulysses Press books call 800-377-2542 or write to Ulysses Press, P.O. Box 3440, Berkeley, CA 94703-3440. All retail orders are shipped free of charge. California residents must include sales tax. Allow two to three weeks for delivery.

ABOUT THE AUTHOR

Art Ulene, M.D. is a Clinical Professor at the University of Southern California School of Medicine. Since 1975, Dr. Ulene has spearheaded the use of television to promote public health. His health reports have aired on the NBC TODAY show, the ABC HOME show, and his syndicated feature, "Feeling Fine," ran regularly on local news broadcasts in over 50 cities. Currently, Dr. Ulene is the Medical Expert on the NBC TODAY show. Additionally, he is the author of numerous books and the producer of several video and audio programs. Dr. Ulene lives in Los Angeles.

NOTES:

NOTES:

NOTES:

NOTES: